Freestyle 2018

The Essential Guide to Sustained Weight Loss

By Sophia Lee

© Copyright 2018 **by –Sophia Lee- All rights reserved**.

This document is geared towards providing exact and reliable information in regards to the topic and issue covered. The publication is sold with the idea that the publisher is not required to render accounting, officially permitted, or otherwise, qualified services. If advice is necessary, legal or professional, a practiced individual in the profession should be ordered.

The author, Sophia Lee, is in no way affiliated with, authorized, maintained, sponsored or endorsed by the Weight Watchers International, Inc or any of its affiliates or subsidiaries

Sophia Lee offers no suggestion that the work presented in this book is "official" or produced or sanctioned by the owner or any licensees of the aforementioned trademarks. Sophia Lee will take all steps necessary to ensure that any usage of trademarked items in no way confuses the audience of this book to its origin. Sophia Lee makes no claim to own any of the copyrights or trademarks related to any of the official Weight Watchers International, Inc products. Names that are displayed in this book may be trademarked and/or copyrighted and are the property of their respective owners.

> - From a Declaration of Principles which was accepted and approved equally by a Committee of the American Bar Association and a Committee of Publishers and Associations.

The information provided herein is stated to be truthful and consistent, in that any liability, in terms of inattention or otherwise, by any usage or abuse of any policies, processes, or directions contained within is the solitary and utter responsibility of the recipient reader. Under no circumstances will any legal responsibility or blame be held against the publisher for any reparation, damages, or monetary loss due to the information herein, either directly or indirectly.

All data and information provided in this book is for informational purposes only. Sophia Lee makes no representations as to accuracy, completeness, current, suitability, or validity of any information in this book & will not be liable for any errors, omissions, or delays in this information or any losses, injuries, or damages arising from its display or use. All information is provided on an as-is basis.

Respective authors own all copyrights not held by the publisher.

The information herein is offered for informational purposes solely, and is universal as so. The presentation of the information is without contract or any type of guarantee assurance.

The trademarks that are used are without any consent, and the publication of the trademark is without permission or backing by the trademark owner. All trademarks and brands within this book are for clarifying purposes only and are owned by the owners themselves, not affiliated with this document.

The author is not a licensed practitioner, physician or medical professional and offers no medical treatment, diagnoses, suggestions or counselling. The information presented herein has not been evaluated by the U.S Food & Drug Administration, and it is not intended to diagnose, treat, cure or prevent any disease. Full medical clearance from a licensed physician should be obtained before beginning or modifying any diet, exercise or lifestyle program, and physician should be informed of all nutritional changes. The author claims no responsibility to any person or entity for any liability, loss, damage or death caused or alleged to be caused directly or indirectly as a result of the use, application or interpretation of the information presented herein.

TABLE OF CONTENTS

Introduction ix

Chapter 1: Freestyle, the Beginning x
    Freestyle; the Principles xi

Chapter 2:   The Freestyle Points System xii
    How Much Am I Likely to Lose? xiii

Chapter 3:   The Freestyle Program xiv
    Counting the Freestyle Points! xiv
    New to Freestyle! xiv
    Get to Know your NO Points Foods xv
    Time for Rollover! xvi
    How Do Rollover Points Work? xvi
    Good News for Existing Members xvi
    Come Dine with Us! xvii

BREAKFAST 1
    Avocado Veggie Egg Scramble 2
    Coco Chia Pudding with Berries and Lime 3
    Country Cottage Pancakes 4
    Dark Chocolate Orange Brunch Scones 5
    Eggs Benedict Flatbreads 6

Make-Ahead Breakfast Muffin Sandwiches 7

Mexican Chilaquiles 8

Oatmeal and Banana Muffins 9

Peanut Butter and Jelly Yogurt Bowl 10

Pumpkin Pie French Toast 11

Strawberry Breakfast Protein Smoothie 12

DESSERT 13

Brown Sugar Streusel French Toast Muffins 14

Blueberry and Lemon Cupcakes 15

Choc Chip Cannoli Tarts 16

Chocolate Peppermint Mini Cheesecakes 17

Coconut Almond Macaroons 18

Coconut Almond Macaroons 19

Dark Chocolate Dipped Strawberries 20

Date and Chocolate Cookie Pie 21

Dutch Baby Mini Pancakes 22

Fruity Spanish Sangria Popsicles 23

Minted Strawberry Sorbet. 24

Strawberry Baked Doughnuts 25

Vanilla Peach Puddings 26

PASTA & GRAINS. 27

Cheddar Beef Taco Pasta 28

Cheddar Cheese and Bacon Risotto with Beer 29

Chicken Lasagna 30

Creamy Pasta Salad with Avocado and Bacon 31

Hot 'n Creamy Chicken Penne 32

Mushroom and Garlic Quinoa 33

Pea and Scallop Linguine 34

Pineapple Fried Rice with Shrimp. 35

Sage and Pumpkin, Sausage Tortellini 36

Tomato Chicken Orzo 37

Winter Greens and Poached Egg Fettuccini 38

POULTRY 39

BBQ Bean and Chicken Bubble Up. 40

Coconut Breaded Chicken Tenders 41

Cordon Bleu Skillet Chicken 42

Feta and Butternut Squash Turkey Skillet 43

Honey and Balsamic Glazed Chicken 44

Moroccan Olive and Chicken Tagine 45

Rustic Leftover Turkey Broccoli Casserole. 46

Shepherd's Pie with Sweet Potato 47

Slow Cooked Chicken with Mushrooms 48

Sweet and Smoky Apricot Chicken 49

Thai Spiced Peanut Chicken 50

RED MEAT. 51

African Harissa Grilled Lamb 52

Bacon Burger Quesadillas 53

Cornflake Crusted Pork Chops 54

Hearty Beef and Barley Casserole 55

Korean Beef Bowls 56

Peach and Ginger Roast Pork Tenderloin 57

Philly Cheesesteak Mushrooms 58

Spicy Pepper Cubed Steak. 59

Swedish Meatballs in Creamy Gravy 60

Sweet Mustard Spiral Ham 61

Zesty Lime and Garlic Pork Chops 62

SEAFOOD 63

Blackened Halibut Tacos with Fruity Slaw 64

Chickpea, Caper, and Tuna Salad 65

Crispy Shrimp Taquitos. 66

Garlic and Herb Tilapia. 67

Grilled Lemon and Salmon Kebabs 68

Hot Crab Salad Stuffed Avocado 69

Lobster Salad with Asparagus 70

Mussels in White Wine and Basil Cream 71

Seared Scallop Tostadas with Homemade Guacamole. 72

Swordfish Steak Burgers. 73

Zucchini Wrapped Cod 74

SNACKS 75

Brownie Batter Fruit Dip 76

Caramel Pretzel Balls 77

Crunchy Cajun Spiced Chickpeas. 78

Frozen Yogurt Candy Buttons. 79

Garlic Breaded Mozzarella Sticks 80

Greek Style Nachos 81

Hawaiian Pizza Cups 82

Homemade Potato Chips 83

Hot 'n Cheesy Buffalo Chicken Dip 84

Parmesan Kale Chips 85

Ranch Style Hummus. 86

SOUPS, STEWS & CHILLIES 87

Fiery Caribbean Chicken Stew 88

Italian Wedding Soup with Meatballs 89

Mexican Chicken Tortilla Soup 90

Mixed Vegetable and Lentil Stew 91

Salmon and Potato Chowder 92

South American Beef and Beer Stew 93

Split Pea and Ham Soup 94

Stracciatella Soup with Spinach and Orzo. 95

Traditional Minestrone Soup 96

Turkey Chilli Soup 97

Vegetable and Pumpkin Chilli 98

VEGGIES & VEGETARIAN 99

Blueberry and Fresh Corn Salad with Lime Honey Dressing 100

Brie and Pear Grilled Cheese Sandwiches. .101

Broccoli Parmigianno 102

Corn and Zucchini Frittata with Cheese 103

Golden Cauliflower Nuggets 104

Indian Potato Cauliflower Curry 105

Lemon Avocado Toast with Chia Seeds 106

Quinoa and Squash Salad with Citrus Dressing 107

Simple Caesar Salad. 108

Vegetable Chow Mein. 109

Vegetable Tots. 110

Take Control & Win the War! .111

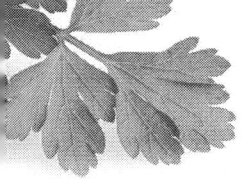

INTRODUCTION

Losing weight needn't be an uphill struggle. You just have to put behind you nearly everything that you have read or learned over the years about weight loss.

The hardened dieters amongst us know that nine times out of ten, we lose weight only to pile it back on again. In fact, often gaining, and in lots of cases, even more, weight than we lost in the first place.

Why is this I hear you ask? Well, quite simply most of the diets we choose are no more than a quick fix. They aren't tailor-made to take into account our age, gender, weight, and height. Diets, like our bodies, don't fit into one-size fits all scenario.

Freestyle understands this and allows you to enjoy the foods you like, and still lose unwanted weight.

Through this book, you will discover how to form a healthy relationship with your body. From this moment on you will make the right food choices. You will learn how to create recipes which will give you a varied weekly menu and keep you feeling full and satisfied.

The Freestyle program will show you how to lose weight and equally as important, keep it off!

SOPHIA LEE

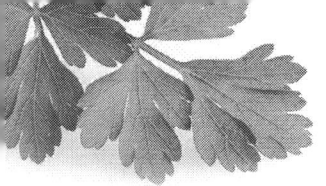

CHAPTER 1

Freestyle, THE BEGINNING

In a 2018 survey by US News, Freestyle achieved the highest score for both overall weight loss and fastest weight loss, with experts hailing the program as being smart and effective.

Pretty impressive, huh? What's more amazing though, is that Freestyle isn't the brainchild of a group of scientists or the money-making initiative of a multi-national corporation.

Freestyle is one woman's answer to overcoming obesity.

We need to travel way back to the early 1960's, a time for mini-skirts, Spiderman and American John Glenn's first orbit of the Earth. While the star of Baby Jane, Bette Davis, was battling it out with Joan Crawford, New York housewife Jean Nidetch was fighting a war of her own, one with her weight.

Jean from Queens, weighing just over 15 stones had always struggled to lose weight. The turning point for her came, however, when one day while shopping she bumped into a neighbor who asked how long before the baby was due.

The 30-year-old housewife ran home, took a long hard look in the mirror and decided enough was enough. She had to do something, and fast.

She went about inviting friends to come together in her home once a week to talk about the best ways to lose weight.

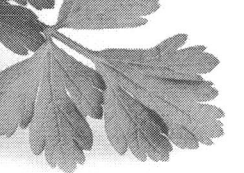

The rest is history, from these humble beginnings, as waists grew smaller and smaller, Freestyle grew bigger and bigger.

Today, it has millions of members all over the world coming together to help achieve their weight loss goals.

Freestyle; the Principles

You will soon discover that Freestyle is like no other weight loss program. It will stress to you the importance of choosing the foods you love to eat. What it won't do, is dictate what you can and can't eat as part of your daily diet.

It believes, just like Jean Nidetch did in those early days, that denying yourself the foods that suit you is not a long-term solution to successful weight loss.

Using the Freestyle Points system, Freestyle will show you how to make healthier, daily and weekly food choices.

The system takes into consideration weekend cravings, special occasions, and times when staying within your Smart Point allowance just isn't a possibility. In other words, Freestyle is a diet for life and one which fits into your lifestyle.

Jean's New York weekly meetings that were so popular, now take place all over the country, and in fact, the world. They are a chance to meet up with and, chat to, other dieters. You will have the opportunity to swap ideas and recipes, and they will give you the support and encouragement that is so vital for those ups and downs.

You will also discover how to incorporate physical activity into your daily life without having to hit the gym too hard – unless of course, you want to!

Freestyle will help you to ditch those negative eating habits and feelings forever.

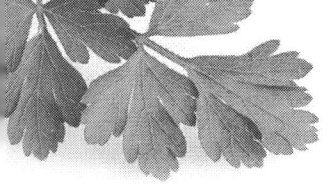

CHAPTER 2
THE Freestyle Points SYSTEM

Count the points and not the Calories!

Did you know that when we count calories, we stop paying attention to the food choices we are making? We no longer look at what we are eating because all we see is a sequence of numbers.

We choose to eat things that are lower in calories rather than the foods we enjoy. Very soon we are on a downward spiral of dissatisfaction. Food cravings kick-in as we deny ourselves the foods we love.

Now, not only are we battling with the scales, we are at war with the calculator.

Freestyle Points take into account protein, sugar, and saturated fat as well as calorific content. The more weight you have to lose, the higher your point allocation.

We calculate for you, based on your age, gender, current weight, and height, the number of points you can enjoy every day, while still losing up to 2 pounds a week.

You 'spend' these points throughout the week and it's totally up to you how what on, and when you spend these points. Plus, you have the option to carry Freestyle Points forward for those special occasions – but more on that later.

Lean protein, fruit, and veggies are NO Points, so very soon and without even realizing it, you will be making healthier food choices.

Foods that are higher in saturated fat and sugar cost more points, but you can still include them if, and when, you want.

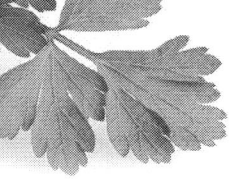

How Much Am I Likely to Lose?

The 64 million dollar question!

In reality, we should be asking how much will I lose and how much of what I lose will I keep off!

Again, it's not a one-size fits all. Bodies have different needs, but the program is designed for you to lose between 1-2 pounds of unwanted weight each week. And providing you follow the system, the pounds won't pile back on either.

You will lose weight responsibly and without any of the nasty side effects of rapid and unhealthy weight loss, such as irritability, extreme tiredness, hair loss, and loose skin. Not to mention long-term and sometimes serious health complications.

So now it's time to not only put away the calculator, but also the weight loss pills, miracle teas, and other fad diet paraphernalia.

Remember, with Freestyle you are losing fat, which unlike water will not pile back on the moment a fork or glass hits your lips!

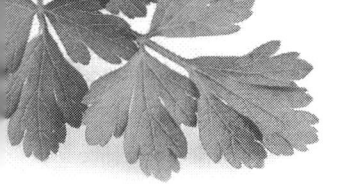

CHAPTER 3
THE FREESTYLE PROGRAM

Counting the Freestyle Points!

You now know that by counting the Freestyle Points you don't have to deny yourself your favorite foods.

Pizza, ice cream, soda, beer or wine are no longer forbidden to you!

From now on, all you have to do is personalize your program to fit in around your life, and rather than feeling guilty, enjoy those foods that give you pleasure.

To help you do just this, you will discover further on in this book, dozens of creative and mouth-watering recipes that will show you how to prepare your favorite foods. What's more, we have calculated the Smart Point value for you too.

New to Freestyle!

If we count Freestyle Points and keep to our point allocation, allowing of course for those special occasions, we are well on the way to winning the battle with unwanted weight.

We also know that the Freestyle Points system is tried tested and achieves proven results.

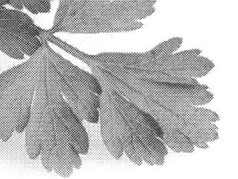

What we haven't talked about yet though, is the new NO Points Foods introduced by Freestyle to give you even more freedom and flexibility.

There are over 200 foods in this category.

Food staples including fish, seafood, chicken, eggs, beans, corn, fruit, and veggies. You can eat these without taking off any points from your daily points budget.

They don't need to be tracked, measured or accounted for, which means you have more time to yes, you guessed it, get on with your life!

As if Free Points weren't enough, Freestyle have recently introduced Rollovers.

Rollovers allow you to, as the name suggests, allow you to carry over Freestyle Points from one day to the next but you will have to wait a little longer to hear more on that!

Get to Know your NO Points Foods

Getting to know your NO Points Foods is the most effective way of getting the most out of the Freestyle program.

These 200 foods will help to fill you up and keep hunger at bay without losing any of your Freestyle Points daily allowance. This is really helpful on those days when you are planning on banking Rollover Points.

Fruit and veggies on the NO Points Foods list can be frozen, fresh or canned. The only requirement is that they have no added oil, sugar or seasoning. You should always prepare them drained.

Meat, poultry, and seafood may be frozen, fresh or canned. As with fruit and veggies, with no added oil, sugar or seasoning and drained.

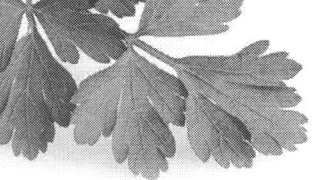

Don't forget, there is need to weigh, measure or count these foods either.

Time for Rollover!

Unlike other weight loss programs, Freestyle takes into account real-life situations. It is these that can jeopardize a diet.

How many times have you kept to a diet all week only to blow it on the weekend? When this happens, it is very easy to go right back to square one and write-off the week. In fact, sometimes it can even result in giving up altogether.

Freestyle understands this dilemma. So now, with the introduction of Rollover Points, there is no need to feel guilty for eating that slice of pie or birthday cake.

How Do Rollover Points Work?

As we now know, Freestyle Points are a weekly budget, and every day there is a limit.

So just like any budget, if you know, there is something out of the ordinary about to happen you can budget for it, bank it, and spend the Rollover Points when you need them.

You can bank up to 4 Freestyle Points every day. On those days all you have to do is simply fill up on those NO Points Foods.

Good News for Existing Members

For anyone already following the Freestyle program, you are well familiarized with Freestyle Points. Maybe you don't know, however, that to allow for the new NO Points foods, your daily points budget will change.

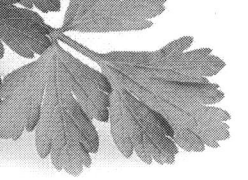

Your new budget will take into account your age, gender, current weight, and height.

You can learn more about this at your weekly meeting, or online.

Come Dine with Us!

It's easy to become bored with the foods we eat, and this is especially so for anyone on a weight loss or management program.

So when boredom kicks in, it's time to move things up a gear and look for a little inspiration.

Our 100 sweet and savory recipes are creative, easy to make, and family friendly.

To make your time in the kitchen stress-free, we have calculated a Smart Point value, cooking time, and portion size for each recipe.

Divided into 9 sections; Breakfasts, Dessert, Pasta & Grains, Poultry, Red Meat, Seafood, and Snacks, Soups, Stews & Chilies, Veggies & Vegetarian, it's a must-have recipe book for anyone following the Freestyle program.

It's time to battle the boredom with Dark Chocolate Orange Brunch Scones, Pumpkin Pie French Toast, Indian Potato Cauliflower Curry, Zesty Lime & Garlic Pork Chops, and Minted Strawberry Sorbet.

Watching your weight never tasted so good!

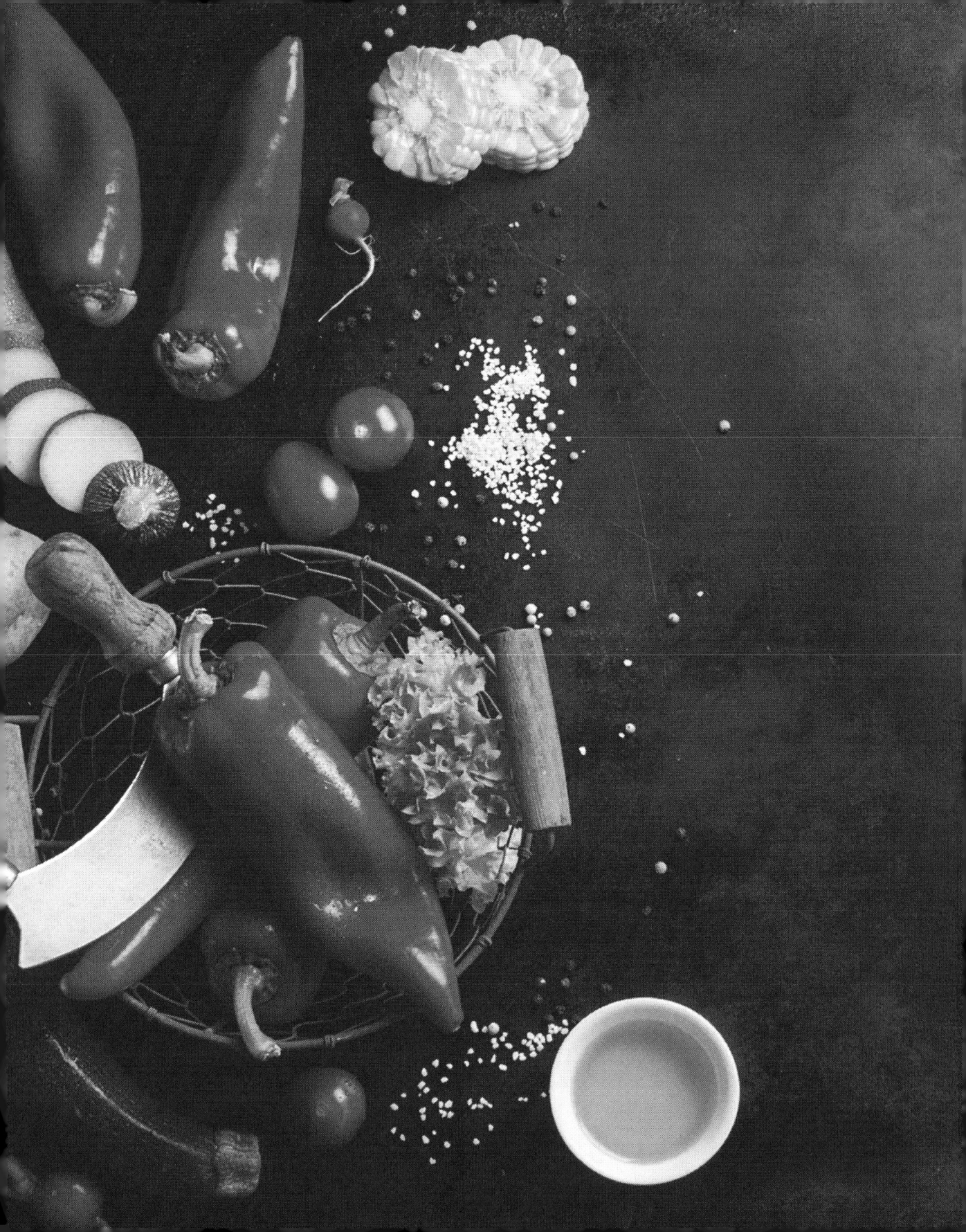

Breakfast

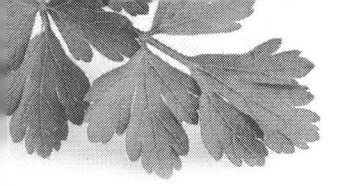

Avocado Veggie Egg Scramble

(Prep Time: 10 MIN | Cook Time: 10 MIN | Serves: 4)

Ingredients:

For cooking:

2 tsp olive oil

For scramble:

1 red bell pepper (seeded, diced)
½ cup red onion (peeled, finely chopped)
2 cups broccoli florets (finely chopped)
8 medium eggs (beaten)
Sea salt and black pepper
1 medium tomato (finely chopped)
1 ripe, medium avocado (peeled, pitted, sliced)

Directions:

1. In a skillet over moderately high heat, sauté the bell pepper, onion, and broccoli in the olive oil for 3-4 minutes.
2. Add the beaten egg and cook, while stirring, until you achieve your desired level of 'doneness.'
3. Divide between four plates and season well with sea salt and black pepper. Top each portion with a little chopped tomato and sliced avocado.

Freestyle Points Per Serving: 4

(Calories 280 | Total Fats 20g | Net Carbs: 6g | Protein 16g | Fiber: 6g)

FREESTYLE 2018

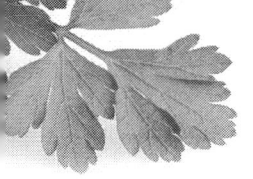

Coco Chia Pudding with Berries and Lime

(Prep Time: 8 HOUR 5 MIN | Cook Time: N/A | Serves: 2)

Ingredients:

For pudding:
½ cup fresh raspberries
6-7 drops liquid stevia sweetener of choice
½ cup canned low-fat coconut milk
2 tbsp chia seeds
½ cup almond coconut milk (unsweetened)
1 tsp lime zest (grated)
1 tbsp shredded coconut (unsweetened)
1 tsp freshly squeezed lime juice

For topping:
¼ cup fresh raspberries
¼ cup fresh strawberries (hulled, chopped)

Directions:

1. Add all pudding ingredients to a re-sealable container, and stir well until combined. Seal with a lid and chill overnight.
2. The following morning, divide between two glasses or bowls and top with equal amounts of fresh raspberries and strawberries.
3. Serve.

Freestyle Points Per Serving: 5

(Calories 155 | Total Fats 10g | Net Carbs: 5g | Protein 4g | Fiber: 10g)

BREAKFAST

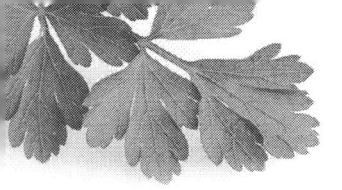

Country Cottage Pancakes

(Prep Time: 10 MIN | Cook Time: 15 MIN | Serves: 4)

Ingredients:

For cooking:
Nonstick spray

For pancakes:
1 cup low-fat cottage cheese
8 medium eggs
4 tbsp almond flour
4 tbsp coconut flour
½ tsp bicarb of soda
1 tsp lemon zest (grated)
Pinch kosher salt
½ tsp vanilla essence
4 tbsp sweetened almond milk

Directions:

1. Add all ingredients (excluding the almond milk) to a blender and blitz until smooth.
2. Spritz a skillet with nonstick spray and place over moderately high heat.
3. Ladle a ¼ cup of batter at a time into the skillet. When the mixture begins to bubble, flip and cook until the bubbles start to pop and the edges are firm and cooked.
4. Repeat with the remaining batter and serve straight away.

Freestyle Points Per Serving: 3

(Calories 265 | Total Fats 15g | Net Carbs: 5g | Protein 23g | Fiber: 3g)

FREESTYLE 2018

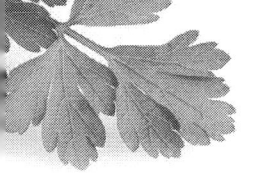

Dark Chocolate Orange Brunch Scones

(Prep Time: 15 MIN | Cook Time: 25 MIN | Serves: 10)

Ingredients:

Orange glaze:
1 tbsp freshly squeezed orange juice
2 tbsp white sugar

Wet ingredients:
½ cup low-fat buttermilk
1 tbsp orange zest (grated)
¼ cup white sugar
1 medium egg
1 tbsp freshly squeezed orange juice

Dry ingredients:
1 cup whole wheat flour
1 cup all-purpose flour
1 tbsp baking powder
3 tbsp salted butter (chilled, chopped)
½ cup dark choc chips

Directions:

1. Preheat the main oven to 375 degrees F and position the rack in the top third of the oven. Line a cookie sheet with parchment and set to one side.
2. Combine the orange glaze ingredients in a small bowl and set to one side.
3. In a second, medium-sized bowl, beat together all of the wet ingredients until combined and set to one side.
4. In a third, large mixing bowl, stir together the flours and baking powder. Using two knives 'cut' in the chopped butter, until mostly incorporated with only very small pieces of butter remaining. Fold in the dark choc chips.
5. Pour the wet ingredients into the butter/flour mixture and stir well until you have a smooth, combined dough.
6. Lightly flour your worktop and turn the scone dough out onto it. Knead the dough four times before transferring it to the cookie sheet. Flatten the dough into a ¾" thick and 8" wide disc. Use a knife to gently score down the center of the dough and divide it into ten equal wedges.
7. Brush the top of the scone dough with the set-aside orange glaze.
8. Place in the oven and bake for just under 20 minutes.
9. Allow to cool to warm before serving.

Freestyle Points Per Serving: 6

(Calories 210 | Total Fats 8g | Net Carbs: 30g | Protein 4g | Fiber: 3g)

BREAKFAST

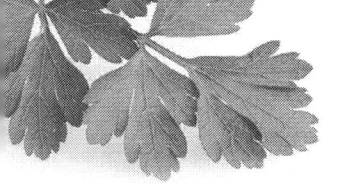

Eggs Benedict Flatbreads

(Prep Time: 15 MIN | Cook Time: 15 MIN | Serves: 4)

Ingredients:

For cooking:
1 tsp olive oil

For sauce:
1 tbsp low-fat mayo
⅓ cup plain non-fat Greek yogurt
½ tbsp freshly squeezed lemon juice
½ tbsp Dijon mustard
1 tsp low-calorie salted butter

For egg flatbreads:
1 tbsp apple cider vinegar
4 medium eggs
4 rashers centre-cut bacon
2 low-calorie grain flatbreads (figure eight shaped, slice in half)
Sea salt and black pepper

Directions:

1. First, poach the eggs. Pour water into a skillet over high heat until halfway full. Add the apple cider vinegar and stir well.
2. When boiling, turn down to a simmer and break the eggs directly into the water, one at a time. Cook for approximately 5 minutes.
3. While the eggs cook, fry the bacon rashers in the oil until cooked. This should take approximately 5-6 minutes.
4. Add all of the sauce ingredients (excluding the butter) to a small bowl and stir very well. Pop in the microwave for 30-40 seconds until warm through, and stir in the butter until it melts.
5. To assemble; arrange one cooked rasher of bacon one each flatbread half, top with a poached egg and lightly season the egg with salt and pepper. Spoon over an equal amount of sauce and serve straight away.

Freestyle Points Per Serving: 3

(Calories 175 | Total Fats 10g | Net Carbs: 6g | Protein 16g | Fiber: 3.5g)

FREESTYLE 2018

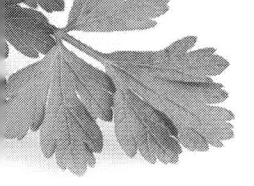

Make-Ahead Breakfast Muffin Sandwiches

(Prep Time: 10 MIN | Cook Time: 15 MIN | Serves: 12)

Ingredients:

For cooking:
Nonstick spray

For sandwiches:
3 cups liquid egg substitute
Kosher salt and black pepper
12 rashers centre-cut bacon
12 lower-calorie English breakfast muffins (halved)
12 low-fat American cheese slices

Directions:

1. Preheat the main oven to 350 degrees F. Spritz a 13x9" baking tray generously with nonstick spray.
2. Pour the egg substitute into the tray and season with kosher salt and black pepper, stir well and place in the oven for 15 minutes until cooked and set.
3. While the eggs cook, fry the rashers of bacon.
4. When the eggs are finished cooking, slice them into 12 equal squares. Set the bacon and eggs aside to cool completely.
5. Fill each muffin with one square of egg, one rasher of bacon, and one slice of cheese.
6. Wrap each muffin tightly in foil and place in a large Ziploc bag. Seal the bag and pop in the freezer for up to 90 days.
7. When ready to serve; allow to thaw at room temperature overnight. The following morning, warm in the microwave for 60-70 seconds and enjoy.

Freestyle Points Per Serving: 4

(Calories 160 | Total Fats 1.5g | Net Carbs: 18g | Protein 16g | Fiber: 6g)

BREAKFAST

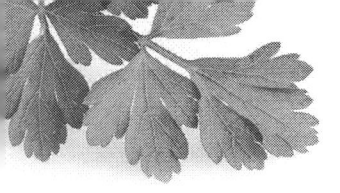

Mexican Chilaquiles

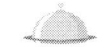 

(Prep Time: 15 MIN | Cook Time: 30 MIN | Serves: 6)

Ingredients:

For cooking:
Nonstick spray

For chilaquiles:
5 (6") low-calorie yellow corn tortillas (sliced into 1"x3" strips)
8 ounces smoked turkey sausage (chopped)
3 cups tomato salsa (chunky)
1 cup fat-free chicken stock
4 ounces low-fat Cheddar cheese (shredded)
1 ripe, medium avocado (peeled, pitted, sliced)
Fresh cilantro (chopped, for garnish)

Directions:

1. Preheat the main oven to 350 degrees F.
2. Arrange the strips of tortilla on a large cookie sheet and spritz evenly with nonstick spray.
3. Place in the oven and bake for 12-14 minutes until crispy. Set to one side.
4. Spritz a skillet with nonstick spray and set over moderate heat. Add the smoked sausage and sauté for 5-6 minutes, until lightly browned. Transfer the sausage to a plate.
5. Using the same skillet, bring the tomato salsa to a simmer. Pour in the chicken stock and stir well. Allow to simmer for 2-3 minutes before returning the smoked sausage to the skillet.
6. Add the cooked tortilla strips to the skillet and stir well. Allow to come to a simmer for 3-4 minutes, until the mixture thickens and the tortillas soften.
7. Take off the heat and scatter with the shredded Cheddar.
8. Arrange the sliced avocado on top and garnish with cilantro.
9. Serve.

Freestyle Points Per Serving: 6

(Calories 235 | Total Fats 12g | Net Carbs: 15g | Protein 15g | Fiber: 6g)

FREESTYLE 2018

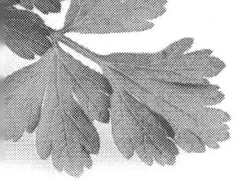

Oatmeal and Banana Muffins

(Prep Time: 10 MIN | Cook Time: 15 MIN | Serves: 9)

Ingredients:

For cooking:
Nonstick spray

For wet ingredients:
2 tbsp canola oil
2 ripe, medium bananas (peeled, mashed)
1 large egg
½ cup skim milk
¾ tsp vanilla essence

For dry ingredients:
1¾ baking powder
½ cup oats (quick cooking variety)
⅔ cup whole wheat flour
¼ cup sugar
Pinch salt
½ tsp cinnamon

Directions:

1. Preheat the main oven to 375 degrees F. Spritz 9 holes of a 12 hole muffin tin with nonstick spray and set to one side.
2. Add all of the wet ingredients to a mixing bowl and beat until combined.
3. To a second mixing bowl, add the dry ingredients and stir well.
4. Fold the dry mixture into the wet mixture, a little at a time, until incorporated.
5. Pour the batter equally into the 9 greased holes. Place in the oven and bake for just over 15 minutes. Allow to cool completely before serving.

Freestyle Points Per Serving: 4

(Calories 130 | Total Fats 4g | Net Carbs: 18.5g | Protein 3.5g | Fiber: 2g)

BREAKFAST

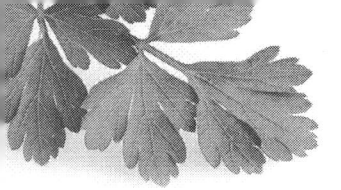

Peanut Butter and Jelly Yogurt Bowl

(Prep Time: 5 MIN | Cook Time: N/A | Serves: 1)

Ingredients:

For yogurt:
6 ounces plain fat-free Greek yogurt
4 tsp low-calorie grape jelly
1 tbsp low-fat peanut butter

For topping:
2 tbsp red grapes (sliced)
1 tsp unsalted peanuts (chopped)

Directions:

1. Add the yogurt to a bowl. Spoon the jelly and peanut butter on top, then gently swirl the three together using a knife.
2. Sprinkle with sliced grapes and chopped peanuts.
3. Enjoy.

Freestyle Points Per Serving: 6

(Calories 240 | Total Fats 7g | Net Carbs: 23g | Protein 22g | Fiber: 1g)

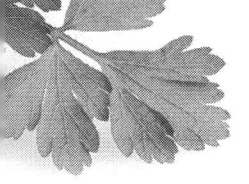

Pumpkin Pie French Toast

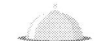

(Prep Time: 10 MIN | Cook Time: 15 MIN | Serves: 5)

Ingredients:

For cooking:
Nonstick spray

For French toast:
½ cup skim milk
3 large eggs
1 tsp pumpkin pie spice
¾ cup canned pureed pumpkin
10 slices low-calorie whole wheat bread

Directions:

1. Add the milk, eggs, pie spice, and canned pumpkin to a shallow dish, whisk well to combine and set to one side.
2. Spritz a skillet with nonstick spray and place over moderately low heat.
3. Dip each slice of bread into the pumpkin mixture and gently press down, this will help the bread soak up the liquid.
4. Cook each slice of soaked bread for a couple of minutes each side, until hot and golden.
5. Serve warm.

Freestyle Points Per Serving: 3

(Calories 145 | Total Fats 4g | Net Carbs: 15g | Protein 10g | Fiber: 7g)

BREAKFAST

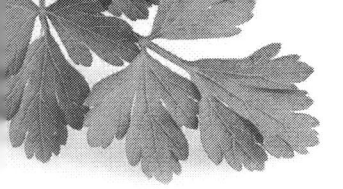

Strawberry Breakfast Protein Smoothie

(Prep Time: 5 MIN | Cook Time: N/A | Serves: 2)

Ingredients:

For smoothie:
1 cup unsweetened almond milk
1 cup plain fat-free Greek yogurt
2 cups fresh strawberries (hulled, chopped)
2 ripe bananas (peeled, chopped)
½ cup oats (quick cooking variety)

Directions:

1. Add all ingredients to a blender and blitz until smooth and lump-free.
2. Pour into two glasses and enjoy straight away*.
   *Enjoy at room temperature for a 'fuller' feeling.

Freestyle Points Per Serving: 4

(Calories 300 | Total Fats 4g | Net Carbs: 49.5g | Protein 3.5g | Fiber: 8g)

FREESTYLE 2018

Dessert

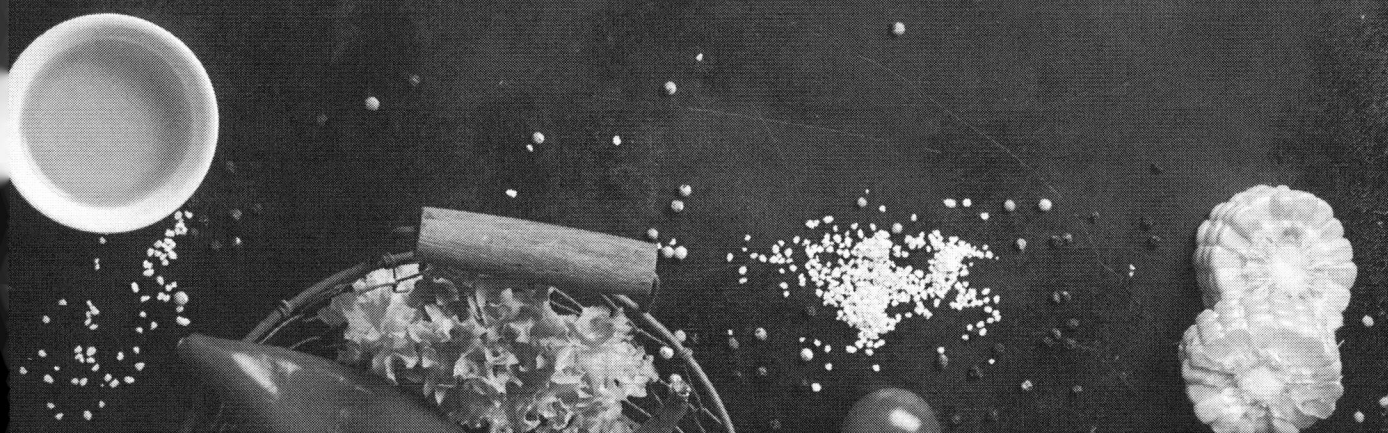

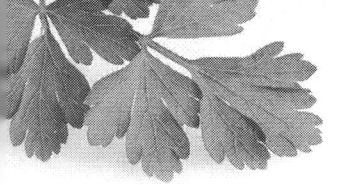

Brown Sugar Streusel French Toast Muffins

(Prep Time: 10 MIN | Cook Time: 25 MIN | Serves: 12)

Ingredients:

For cooking:
Nonstick spray

Wet mixture:
1¼ cups skim milk
3 medium eggs
2 medium egg whites
2 tbsp sugar
2 tsp vanilla essence
1½ tsp ground cinnamon

Dry mixture:
12 slices low-fat whole wheat bread (cut into cubes)
1 apple (peeled, cored, diced)

For streusel topping:
2 tbsp flour
2 tbsp low-fat butter
2 tbsp brown sugar
Pinch kosher salt

Directions:

1. Preheat the main oven to 350 degrees F. Spritz a 12 hole muffin tin with nonstick spray and set to one side.
2. Whisk the ingredients for the wet mixture together in a medium-sized bowl.
3. Toss in the bread cubes and gently press down to help them soak up the liquid. Stir in the diced apple. Spoon the batter equally into the muffin tin.
4. In a second bowl, add the streusel topping ingredients. Using clean fingers, rub the butter into the flour until you have a crumbly mixture.
5. Sprinkle the mixture equally on top of the muffin batter.
6. Place in the oven and bake for just under half an hour. Allow to cool to warm before serving.

Freestyle Points Per Serving: 3

(Calories 116 | Total Fats 3g | Net Carbs: 15g | Protein 6g | Fiber: 3g)

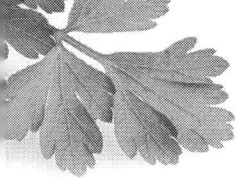

Blueberry and Lemon Cupcakes

(Prep Time: 15 MIN | Cook Time: 25 MIN | Serves: 24)

Ingredients:

For cooking:

Nonstick spray

Lemon blueberry mixture:

½ cup low-fat buttermilk

3½ tbsp freshly squeezed lemon juice

1½ tsp lemon zest (grated)

2 cups fresh blueberries

Wet mixture:

3 tbsp applesauce (unsweetened)

3 tbsp salted butter (at room temperature)

5 ounces low-fat cream cheese (at room temperature)

½ tsp vanilla essence

1½ cups sugar

2 large eggs

Whites of 2 large eggs

Directions:

1. Preheat the main oven to 350 degrees F. Spritz two, 12 hole cupcake tins with nonstick spray.
2. First, make the wet mixture. Beat together the applesauce, butter, and cream cheese until fluffy.
3. Add the vanilla, sugar, eggs, and whites; beat again until combined. Set to one side for a moment.
4. In a second bowl, combine the ingredients for the dry mixture.
5. Using an electric whisk, mix the dry mixture into the wet cream cheese mixture until combined.
6. Add the buttermilk, lemon juice, and zest. Whisk until incorporated.
7. Fold in the blueberries.
8. Spoon the batter into the cupcake tins.
9. Place in the oven and bake for just under half an hour. Allow to cool completely before serving.

Freestyle Points Per Serving: 5

(Calories 135 | Total Fats 4g | Net Carbs: 22g | Protein 3g | Fiber: 1g)

DESSERT

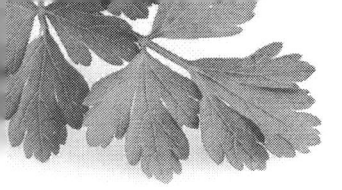

Choc Chip Cannoli Tarts

(Prep Time: 10 MIN | Cook Time: N/A | Serves: 15)

Ingredients:

For cannoli filling:

⅔ cup fat-free ricotta cheese
2 ounces mascarpone cheese
3 tbsp confectioner's sugar
⅛ tsp ground cinnamon
¼ tsp vanilla essence
⅔ cup milk choc chips

For tarts:

15 mini phyllo pastry shells
⅓ cup dark choc chips

Directions:

1. First, make the cannoli filling; beat together the cheeses, sugar, cinnamon, and vanilla essence until fluffy.
2. Fold in the milk choc chips.
3. Spoon the filling mixture equally into the phyllo shells. Scatter the tarts with more dark choc chips.
4. Enjoy straight away or chill until ready to serve.

Freestyle Points Per Serving: 3

(Calories 65 | Total Fats 3g | Net Carbs: 7g | Protein 2g | Fiber: 0g)

FREESTYLE 2018

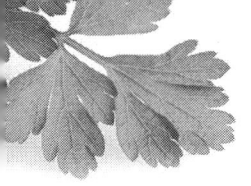

Chocolate Peppermint Mini Cheesecakes

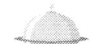

(Prep Time: 2 HOUR 10 MIN | Cook Time: 20 MIN | Serves: 12)

Ingredients:

For cheesecakes:

- 12 low-fat chocolate wafer biscuits
- 8 ounces low-fat cream cheese (at room temperature)
- 1 (5.3 ounce) container vanilla flavored fat-free Greek yogurt
- ⅓ cup white sugar
- 1 large egg
- ¼ tsp peppermint essence

For topping:

- 12 tbsp non-fat whip topping
- 3 mini candy canes (crushed)

Directions:

1. Preheat the main oven to 375 degrees F. Line a 12 hole cupcake tin with liners.
2. Place a chocolate wafer in the base of each cupcake liner. You may need to break the wafers into smaller pieces to make them fit.
3. Add all remaining cheesecake ingredients to a medium-sized bowl and beat until combined. Spoon the mixture equally into the liners on top of the wafers.
4. Place in the oven and bake for just over 15 minutes.
5. Allow to cool completely before chilling for 2 hours.
6. Top each mini cheesecake with 1 tbsp of whip topping and a sprinkling of crushed candy cane.

Freestyle Points Per Serving: 5

(Calories 116 | Total Fats 5g | Net Carbs: 14g | Protein 3g | Fiber: 0g)

DESSERT

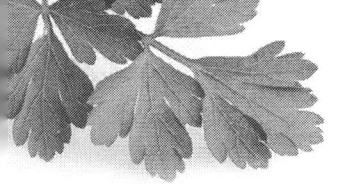

Coconut Almond Macaroons

(Prep Time: 40 MIN | Cook Time: 45 MIN | Serves: 17)

Ingredients:

For cooking:
Nonstick spray

For macaroons:
⅔ cup white sugar
Whites of 5 large eggs
10 ounces flaked coconut (sweetened)
¼ tsp vanilla essence
½ tsp almond essence
Pinch kosher salt

Directions:

1. Cover a cookie sheet with parchment paper and spritz with nonstick spray. Set to one side.
2. Add the sugar, egg whites, and flaked coconut to a saucepan over moderately low heat. Cook, while stirring, for approximately 12 minutes until the ingredients are moist and sticky.
3. Take off the heat and stir in the essences and kosher salt.
4. Chill the mixture for half an hour.
5. Preheat the main oven to 300 degrees F.
6. Drop tablespoonfuls of the mixture onto the cookie sheet to make 34 macaroons.
7. Place in the oven and bake for just under half an hour.
8. Allow to cool completely before serving.

Freestyle Points Per Serving: 6

(Calories 130 | Total Fats 7g | Net Carbs: 13.5g | Protein 2g | Fiber: 1g)

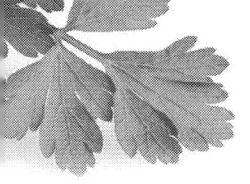

Coconut Almond Macaroons

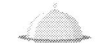

(Prep Time: 40 MIN | Cook Time: 45 MIN | Serves: 17)

Ingredients:

For cooking:
Nonstick spray

For macaroons:
⅔ cup white sugar
Whites of 5 large eggs
10 ounces flaked coconut (sweetened)
¼ tsp vanilla essence
½ tsp almond essence
Pinch kosher salt

Directions:

1. Cover a cookie sheet with parchment paper and spritz with nonstick spray. Set to one side.
2. Add the sugar, egg whites, and flaked coconut to a saucepan over moderately low heat. Cook, while stirring, for approximately 12 minutes until the ingredients are moist and sticky.
3. Take off the heat and stir in the essences and kosher salt.
4. Chill the mixture for half an hour.
5. Preheat the main oven to 300 degrees F.
6. Drop tablespoonfuls of the mixture onto the cookie sheet to make 34 macaroons.
7. Place in the oven and bake for just under half an hour.
8. Allow to cool before serving.

Freestyle Points Per Serving: 6

(Calories 130 | Total Fats 7g | Net Carbs: 13.5g | Protein 2g | Fiber: 1g)

DESSERT

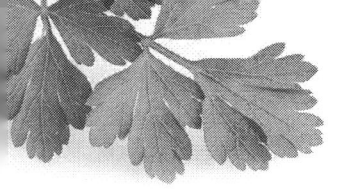

Dark Chocolate Dipped Strawberries

(Prep Time: 30 MIN | Cook Time: 2 MIN | Serves: 18)

Ingredients:

For dipped strawberries:
2 ounces dark chocolate candy melts
18 fresh, large strawberries

Directions:

1. Cover a cookie sheet with parchment paper and set to one side.
2. Add the candy melts to a medium-sized bowl and melt in the microwave in 30-second bursts. Stir until glossy.
3. Use the stems to dip each strawberry in the melted chocolate and then place on the cookie sheet.
4. Chill for 15-20 minutes, until the chocolate has set, before serving.

Freestyle Points Per Serving: 2

(Calories 40 | Total Fats 2g | Net Carbs: 4g | Protein 0g | Fiber: 1g)

FREESTYLE 2018

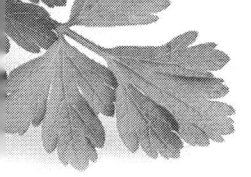

Date and Chocolate Cookie Pie

(Prep Time: 10 MIN | Cook Time: 35 MIN | Serves: 14)

Ingredients:

For cooking:
Nonstick spray

For cookie pie:
2 cups dates (pitted)
⅔ cup almond milk (unsweetened)
17½ ounces canned white beans
1 cup oats (quick cooking variety)
¼ cup applesauce (unsweetened)
3 tbsp coconut oil
2 tsp vanilla essence
½ tsp bicarb of soda
2 tsp baking powder
¼ tsp kosher salt
1 cup dark choc chips

Directions:

1. Preheat the main oven to 350 degrees F. Spritz a 10" springform cake tin with nonstick spray.
2. Add all cookie pie ingredients to a food processor (excluding the dark choc chips) and blitz until smooth.
3. Stir in the dark choc chips until incorporated.
4. Press the cookie dough into the prepared tin.
5. Place in the oven and bake for just over 35 minutes until firm.
6. Allow to cool until just warm before slicing into 14 wedges and serving.

Freestyle Points Per Serving: 5

(Calories 225 | Total Fats 9g | Net Carbs: 34g | Protein 3g | Fiber: 6g)

DESSERT

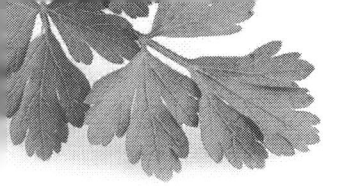

Dutch Baby Mini Pancakes

(Prep Time: 10 MIN | Cook Time: 15 MIN | Serves: 12)

Ingredients:

For cooking:
Nonstick spray

For pancakes:
6 medium eggs
1 cup non-fat milk
¼ cup salted butter (melted)
1 cup all-purpose flour
1 tsp lemon zest (grated)
1 tsp vanilla essence
Pinch kosher salt

Directions:

1. Preheat the main oven to 400 degrees F. Spritz two, 12 hole muffin tins with nonstick spray.
2. Add all pancake ingredients to a blender and blitz until combined.
3. Pour the batter equally into the muffin tins.
4. Place in the oven for just over 12 minutes until golden and puffed up.
5. Top with your favorite Zero Point fruits or non-fat yogurt and serve.

Freestyle Points Per Serving: 3

(Calories 110 | Total Fats 7g | Net Carbs: 6g | Protein 5g | Fiber: 1g)

FREESTYLE 2018

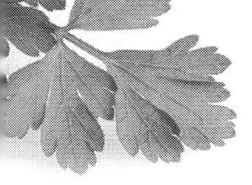

Fruity Spanish Sangria Popsicles

(Prep Time: 8 HOUR 25 MIN | Cook Time: 2 MIN | Serves: 6)

Ingredients:

For fruit mixture:

½ cup apple (peeled, diced)
½ orange (peeled, diced)
¾ cup Spanish dry red wine

For juice mixture:

¾ cup low-calorie orange juice
3 tbsp granulated sugar
Juice of 1 large lemon

Directions:

1. Add the fruit to a bowl and pour over the wine. Set aside for 15 minutes to soak.
2. In a second bowl, add all juice mixture ingredients and stir to combine. Microwave for 90-100 seconds, removing at intervals to stir, until the sugar has melted. Set aside to cool.
3. Add the juice mixture to the soaked fruit and stir to combine.
4. Pour the mixture equally into 6 popsicle molds and freeze overnight.

Freestyle Points Per Serving: 3

(Calories 65 | Total Fats 0g | Net Carbs: 11g | Protein 0g | Fiber: 1g)

DESSERT

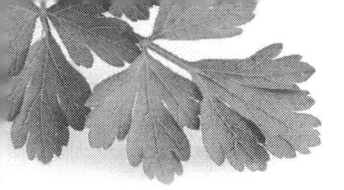

Minted Strawberry Sorbet

(Prep Time: 6 HOUR 10 MIN | Cook Time: N/A | Serves: 5)

Ingredients:

For sorbet:

1 pound fresh, sweet strawberries (washed, hulled)

Juice of 1 medium lime

¼ cup fresh mint (finely chopped)

⅓ cup sugar

Directions:

1. Add all ingredients to a food processor and blitz until combined and smooth.
2. Transfer the mixture to an ice cream maker. Churn and freeze according to manufacturer's directions.
3. Allow to stand at room temperature for a few minutes before scooping and serving.

Freestyle Points Per Serving: 5

(Calories 85 | Total Fats 0g | Net Carbs: 20g | Protein 1g | Fiber: 2g)

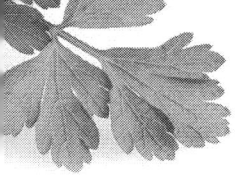

Strawberry Baked Doughnuts

(Prep Time: 15 MIN | Cook Time: 8 MIN | Serves: 6)

Ingredients:

For cooking:

Nonstick spray

For doughnuts:

⅓ cup fresh strawberries (hulled, diced)
1 tbsp pure maple syrup
⅓ cup granulated sugar
1 cup all-purpose flour
½ tsp kosher salt
¼ tsp ground cinnamon
1 tsp baking powder
1 medium egg
⅓ cup skim milk
1 tbsp salted butter (melted)

Directions:

1. Preheat the main oven to 425 degrees F. Spritz a 6-hole donut tin with nonstick spray and set to one side.
2. Add the strawberries to a bowl and pour over the maple syrup. Toss to combine.
3. Add the sugar, flour, salt, cinnamon, and baking powder in a mixing bowl and stir well.
4. Mix the egg, milk, and melted butter into the flour mixture until incorporated.
5. Fold in the strawberries.
6. Divide the mixture equally between the holes in the donut tin.
7. Place in the oven and bake for several minutes until cooked in the centre.
8. Allow to cool completely before serving.

Freestyle Points Per Serving: 6

(Calories 200 | Total Fats 3g | Net Carbs: 36g | Protein 4g | Fiber: 2g)

DESSERT

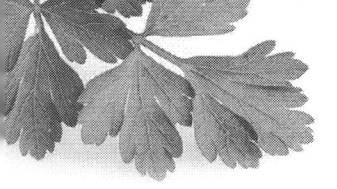

Vanilla Peach Puddings

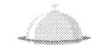

(Prep Time: 2 HOUR 10 MIN | Cook Time: 2 MIN | Serves: 6)

Ingredients:

For puddings:
1 (0.3 ounce) sachet sugar-free peach flavor jello powder
1 pound vanilla flavored non-fat Greek yogurt
⅓ cup peaches (peeled, finely chopped)
12 tbsp non-fat whip topping

Directions:

1. Line a 6 holes of a 12 hole muffin tin with liners and set to one side for a moment.
2. Add the jello powder and yogurt to a medium-sized bowl and stir until combined.
3. Heat in the microwave for a few minutes, removing at intervals to stir, until the peach jello has dissolved.
4. Fold in the chopped peach until evenly distributed.
5. Spoon the mixture evenly into the 6 liners. Transfer to the refrigerator for 2 hours.
6. Top each pudding with 2 tbsp of whip topping before serving.

Freestyle Points Per Serving: 2

(Calories 65 | Total Fats 1g | Net Carbs: 5g | Protein 7g | Fiber: 0g)

Pasta & Grains

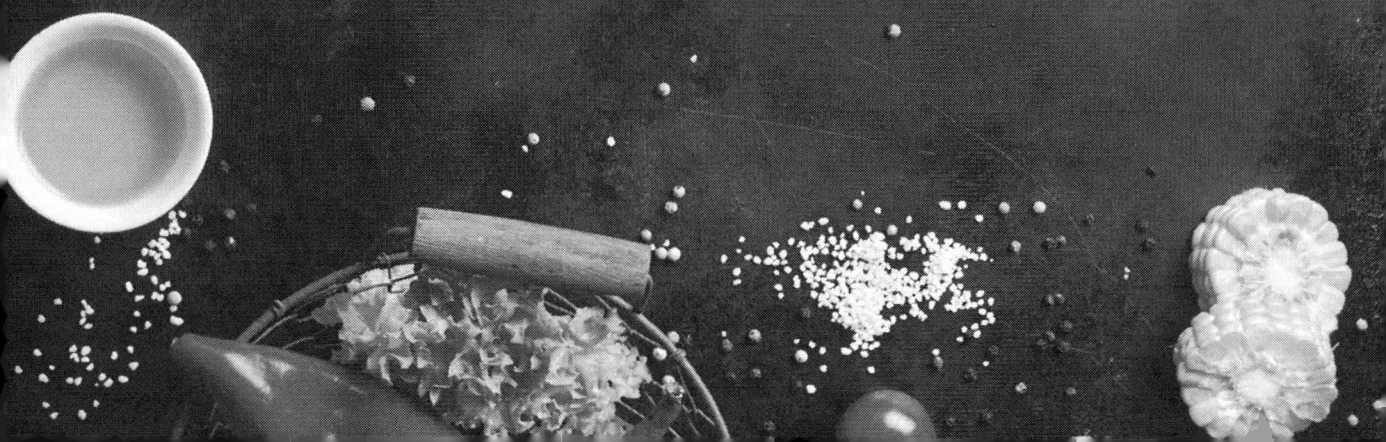

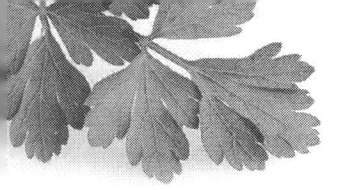

Cheddar Beef Taco Pasta

(Prep Time: 15 MIN | Cook Time: 20 MIN | Serves: 6)

Ingredients:

For pasta:

8 ounces wheat pasta
1 pound 95% lean ground beef
1 (1 ounce) sachet reduced--salt taco seasoning mix
1½ cups chunky salsa
½ cup cold water
¼ cup fat-free sour cream
¾ cup low-fat Cheddar cheese (shredded)
¾ cup sharp Cheddar cheese (shredded)
Salt and pepper (to taste)

Directions:

1. Cook the pasta according to the package directions
2. In the meantime, and while the pasta cooks, add the ground beef to a frying pan and over moderately high heat, using a wooden spoon break the meat up, cook until browned all over.
3. Drain the grease from the pan and add the taco seasoning mix, chunky salsa, and water. Reduce the heat, and simmer until the pasta has finished cooking, for approximately 4-5 minutes.
4. As soon as the pasta is cooked, drain and add it to the beef. Pour in the sour cream, and add the cheese. Season with salt and pepper and stir to incorporate.
5. When the cheese has melted, remove from the heat and serve.

Freestyle Points Per Serving: 10

(Calories 376 | Total Fats 13g | Net Carbs: 31g | Protein 29g | Fiber: 6g)

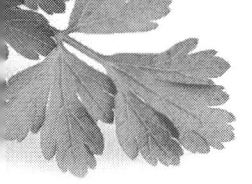

Cheddar Cheese and Bacon Risotto with Beer

(Prep Time: 15 MIN | Cook Time: 30 MIN | Serves: 8)

Ingredients:

For cooking:

1 tbsp low-calorie butter

For risotto:

½ yellow onion (peeled, finely chopped)
2 cloves garlic (peeled, minced)
2 cups Arborio rice
1 (12 ounce) bottle beer of choice
6 cups fat-free chicken stock
4 rashers extra lean turkey bacon (cooked, finely chopped)
1½ ounces Parmesan cheese (finely grated)
⅔ cup low-fat Cheddar cheese (shredded)
¼ tsp cayenne pepper

Directions:

1. In a large pan over moderately high heat, melt the butter.
2. Add the onion to the pan and sauté for 3-4 minutes. Add the minced garlic and cook for another 60 seconds.
3. Add the Arborio rice and cook, while stirring, for 2-3 minutes.
4. Pour in the beer and increase the temperature to high.
5. As the beer starts to simmer, turn the heat down to moderately low and pour in just half a cup of the chicken stock.
6. As soon as the stock has been absorbed, pour in another half a cup. Repeat this process until all of the stock has been used, the mixture is creamy, and the rice is al dente.
7. Take off the heat and sprinkle with the cooked bacon, cheeses, and cayenne pepper. Stir well until the cheeses melt into the risotto.
8. Serve.

Freestyle Points Per Serving: 10

(Calories 280 | Total Fats 7g | Net Carbs: 41g | Protein 10g | Fiber: 0g)

PASTA & GRAINS

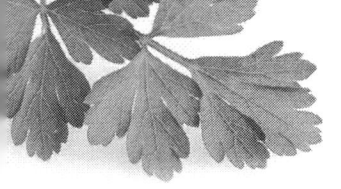

Chicken Lasagna

(Prep Time: 30 MIN | Cook Time: 1 HOUR 10 MIN | Serves: 10)

Ingredients:

For cooking:
Nonstick spray

For lasagna:
2 (25 ounce) jars marinara sauce
1 (8 ounce) package no-boil lasagne noodles
15 ounces fresh low-fat ricotta cheese
2¼ cups low-fat mozzarella cheese (shredded)
3 cups cooked rotisserie chicken (chopped)

Directions:

1. Preheat the main oven to 375 degrees F. Spritz a 9x13" casserole dish with nonstick spray.
2. First, spread around 1 cup of marinara sauce in the base of the dish. Top with a third of the noodles in one single layer. Follow, by spreading all of the ricotta cheese evenly over the top of the noodles.
3. On top of the ricotta cheese, scatter 1 cup of mozzarella cheese, 1½ cups of the chopped chicken and another cup of marinara sauce.
4. Arrange the second third of the noodles in a single layer, top with the remaining chicken and another cup of shredded cheese.
5. Finish with a layer of noodles and pour over any remaining marinara sauce.
6. Cover the baking dish with aluminum foil and bake in the preheated oven for 60 minutes.
7. Remove the foil and top with the remaining shredded cheese. Return to the oven for another several minutes, or until the cheese is totally melted.
8. Remove the dish from the oven and set aside to rest 5-7 minutes.
9. Slice into ten even portions and serve.

Freestyle Points Per Serving: 7

(Calories 350 | Total Fats 10g | Net Carbs: 32g | Protein 27g | Fiber: 4g)Bottom of Form

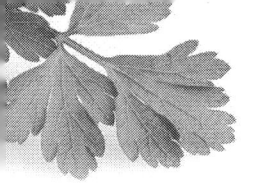

Creamy Pasta Salad with Avocado and Bacon

(Prep Time: 10 MIN | Cook Time: N/A | Serves: 8)

Ingredients:

For pasta salad:
4 cups cooked pasta (preferably corkscrew-shaped)
8 rashers cooked centre-cut bacon (diced)
1 cup cherry tomatoes (quartered)
2 cups romaine lettuce (shredded)

For dressing:
1 ripe, medium avocado (peeled, pitted, mashed)
1½ tsp freshly squeezed lemon juice
¼ cup low-fat mayo
1½ tsp apple cider vinegar
¼ tsp kosher salt
¼ tsp powdered garlic

Directions:

1. Add the pasta salad ingredients to a serving bowl, toss to combine and set to one side for a moment.
2. In a smaller bowl, add all of the dressing ingredients and whisk with a fork until smooth and combined.
3. Pour the dressing over the cooked pasta, gently toss until coated.
4. Keep chilled until ready to serve, enjoy at room temperature.

Freestyle Points Per Serving: 5

(Calories 175 | Total Fats 6g | Net Carbs: 22g | Protein 6g | Fiber: 3g)

PASTA & GRAINS

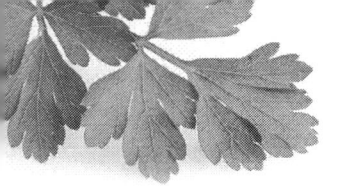

Hot 'n Creamy Chicken Penne

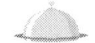

(Prep Time: 10 MIN | Cook Time: 35 MIN | Serves: 8)

Ingredients:

For cooking:
Nonstick spray

For topping:
½ cup low-fat sharp Cheddar cheese

For pasta:
12 ounces penne pasta
2 cup chicken (shredded)
8 ounces fat-free cream cheese
½ cup hot sauce
1 (1 ounce) package ranch seasoning mix
½ cup fat-free sour cream
½ cup low-fat Cheddar cheese

Directions:

1. Preheat the main oven to 375 degrees F. Using nonstick spray, lightly spritz a 9x13" casserole dish and set to one side.
2. Cook the pasta according to the package directions, drain.
3. Combine the drained, cooked penne with the remaining pasta ingredients stirring gently until well combined. Transfer to a casserole dish and evenly spread.
4. Scatter the sharp Cheddar over the top and bake in the preheated oven for just under 20 minutes, or until the cheese melts.

Freestyle Points Per Serving: 6

(Calories 270 | Total Fats 10g | Net Carbs: 18.5g | Protein 20.5g | Fiber: 2g)Bottom of Form

FREESTYLE 2018

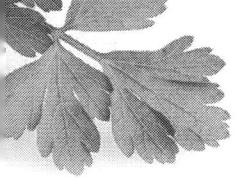

Mushroom and Garlic Quinoa

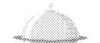 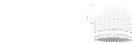

(Prep Time: 5 MIN | Cook Time: 5 HOUR 15 MIN | Serves: 6)

Ingredients:

For quinoa:
- 4 cups vegetable broth
- 2 cups quinoa (uncooked)
- 4 green onions (chopped)
- 12 ounces mushrooms (sliced)
- 4 ounces low-fat cream cheese
- 4 cloves garlic (peeled, minced)
- 1 tsp Italian seasoning
- 1½ tsp sea salt
- 1 tsp black pepper
- ½ cup Parmesan cheese (freshly grated)

Directions:
1. Add all of the ingredients, apart from the freshly grated Parmesan cheese to your slow cooker. Stir to combine.
2. On low heat, cook for 4-5 hours, until the quinoa is cooked through.
3. Scatter with the Parmesan and close the lid of the slow cooker, cook for another 15 minutes, until the cheese is totally melted.

Freestyle Points Per Serving: 8

(Calories 310 | Total Fats 9g | Net Carbs: 39g | Protein 15g | Fiber: 5g) Bottom of Form

PASTA & GRAINS

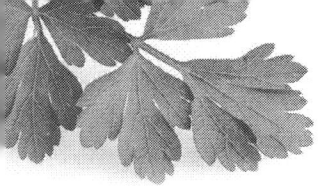

Pea and Scallop Linguine

(Prep Time: 10 MIN | Cook Time: 15 MIN | Serves: 2)

Ingredients:

For cooking:
1 tbsp salted butter

For pasta:
4 ounces whole wheat linguine
1 cup frozen petit pois
2 tbsp fresh parsley (chopped)
1 tsp good-quality olive oil
Sea salt and black pepper
6 large fresh scallops

Directions:

1. Cook the linguine in a deep pot of salted water according to packet directions. Four minutes before the pasta is due to finish cooking, add the petit pois to the water.
2. Drain the pasta and peas, reserving half a cup of the cooking liquid. Return the drained pasta to the pot along with the reserved cooking liquid, parsley, and olive oil. Taste and season with sea salt and black pepper as necessary.
3. While the pasta cooks, prepare the scallops.
4. Melt the butter in a skillet over moderate heat. Add the scallops and cook for 2 and a half minutes on one side, before flipping and cooking for another 40-50 seconds on the other side. The scallops should be opaque throughout.
5. Divide the cooked pasta between two bowls and top each with an equal amount of scallops. Serve straight away.

Freestyle Points Per Serving: 7

(Calories 375 | Total Fats 7g | Net Carbs: 47g | Protein 27g | Fiber: 9g)

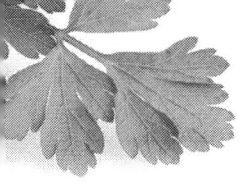

Pineapple Fried Rice with Shrimp

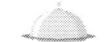

(Prep Time: 10 MIN | Cook Time: 15 MIN | Serves: 4)

Ingredients:

For cooking:

1 tsp olive oil

For fried rice:

1½ cups brown rice
1¼ pounds fresh shrimp (peeled, deveined, chopped)
1 jalapeno (seeded, finely chopped)
3 garlic cloves (peeled, minced)
5 scallions (sliced)
1½ cups pineapple (peeled, chopped)
1 tbsp fish sauce
2 tsp soy sauce
Fresh cilantro (chopped, for garnish)

Directions:

1. Cook the brown rice using packet instructions. Set to one side to cool.
2. Add the oil to a wok and place over high heat.
3. Add the chopped shrimp and sauté for 3-4 minutes until nearly fully-cooked. Transfer the shrimp to a plate.
4. In the same skillet, add the jalapeno, garlic, and scallions. Cook for 60 seconds before adding the chopped pineapple and cooked rice. Stir 3-4 times
5. Add the fish sauce and soy sauce, stir well to combine and cook for a final 30 seconds.
6. Spoon into bowls and garnish with fresh cilantro.

Freestyle Points Per Serving: 8

(Calories 367 | Total Fats 4g | Net Carbs: 56g | Protein 24g | Fiber: 3g)

PASTA & GRAINS

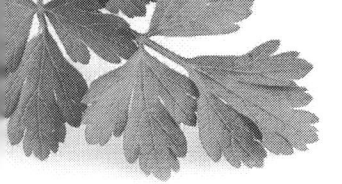

Sage and Pumpkin, Sausage Tortellini

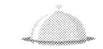 

(Prep Time: 10 MIN | Cook Time: 20 MIN | Serves: 8)

Ingredients:

For pasta:

1 pound Italian hot turkey sausage (without casings)
2 cloves garlic (peeled, minced)
1 yellow onion (peeled, diced)
1 cup fat-free chicken stock
1 cup canned pureed pumpkin
1 (15 ounce) jar reduced-calorie alfredo sauce
20 ounces fresh cheese-filled tortellini (chilled)
5 ounces spinach (chopped)

Seasoning:

¼ tsp black pepper
¼ tsp kosher salt
Pinch cayenne pepper
¼ tsp sage (rubbed)
¼ tsp marjoram

Directions:

1. In a skillet over moderate heat, cook the sausage for 3-4 minutes until browned. Use a wooden spoon to try to break the sausage meat apart as it cooks.
2. Add the garlic and onion and cook, while stirring, until the onions are soft; approximately 3-4 minutes.
3. Pour in the chicken stock, canned pumpkin, Alfredo sauce, and seasoning. Stir very well to combine.
4. Add the cheese tortellini and stir again to coat the pasta in the sauce.
5. Cover the skillet with a lid and gradually increase the heat until you can hear that the sauce is bubbling.
6. Allow to cook at a simmer for several minutes.
7. Uncover the skillet, toss in the spinach and stir until the spinach has wilted.
8. Spoon into bowls and serve straight away.

Freestyle Points Per Serving: 10

(Calories 330 | Total Fats 10g | Net Carbs: 37g | Protein 20g | Fiber: 3g)

FREESTYLE 2018

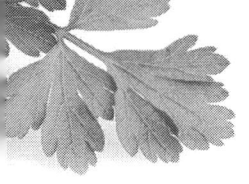

Tomato Chicken Orzo

(Prep Time: 20 MIN | Cook Time: 7 HOUR | Serves: 8)

Ingredients:

For cooking:
Nonstick spray

For chicken:
1 pound boneless chicken breasts
1½ cups chicken broth
2 tbsp garlic salt
1 tbsp freshly ground black pepper

For pasta:
1 (8 ounce) package orzo
2 tsp garlic (minced)
24 grape tomatoes (halved)
4 tbsp Parmesan cheese (freshly grated)

Directions:

1. Add all of the chicken ingredients to your slow cooker and on low, cook for several hours.
2. Approximately half an hour before the chicken is cooked, cook the orzo according to the package instructions.
3. Once the chicken is sufficiently cooked, remove, shred, and set to one side.
4. In the meantime, place a small sauté pan over moderate heat. Add the garlic followed by the tomatoes. Cook until the grape tomatoes burst.
5. Drain the orzo and add to a serving bowl along with the shredded chicken, garlic, and tomatoes. Toss gently until well combined.
6. Scatter with the Parmesan cheese and stir to combine. Serve.

Freestyle Points Per Serving: 4

(Calories 250 | Total Fats 8g | Net Carbs: 23g | Protein 18.5g | Fiber: 1.5g)

PASTA & GRAINS

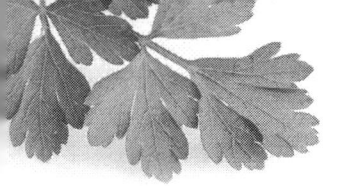

Winter Greens and Poached Egg Fettuccini

(Prep Time: 15 MIN | Cook Time: 20 MIN | Serves: 2)

Ingredients:

For pasta:

- 4 ounces egg fettuccini
- 2 large eggs
- ½ red onion (thinly sliced)
- Sea salt
- 1 garlic clove (peeled, chopped)
- 1 sprig thyme (leaves stripped)
- 4 ounces winter greens of choice (chopped)
- Black pepper

For cooking:

- ½ tbsp olive oil

Directions:

1. Add the pasta to a medium-sized pot of boiling, salted water and cook according to the package instructions. Drain the pasta, setting one cup of the pasta cooking water aside.
2. In the meantime, poach the eggs and drain on kitchen paper towels.
3. While the pasta and poached eggs are cooking, place a pan over moderately high heat.
4. Add the red onion and a pinch of salt to the pan, sauté in olive oil for 3-4 minutes, until they begin to caramelize.
5. Add the garlic and thyme and cook, while stirring, for 60 seconds.
6. Add the winter greens along with ¾ of a cup of the reserved pasta water.
7. Bring to boil, before reducing to a simmer. Cook until the greens are fork tender, this will take 2-3 minutes.
8. Stir in the drained pasta and cook until heated through; 60 seconds.
9. Take the pan off the heat and season to taste.
10. Divide the pasta between two bowls.
11. Top each bowl of pasta with a poached egg. Dust with black pepper and serve.

Freestyle Points Per Serving: 7

(Calories 342 | Total Fats 9g | Net Carbs: 46g | Protein 16g | Fiber: 5g)Bottom of Form

FREESTYLE 2018

Poultry

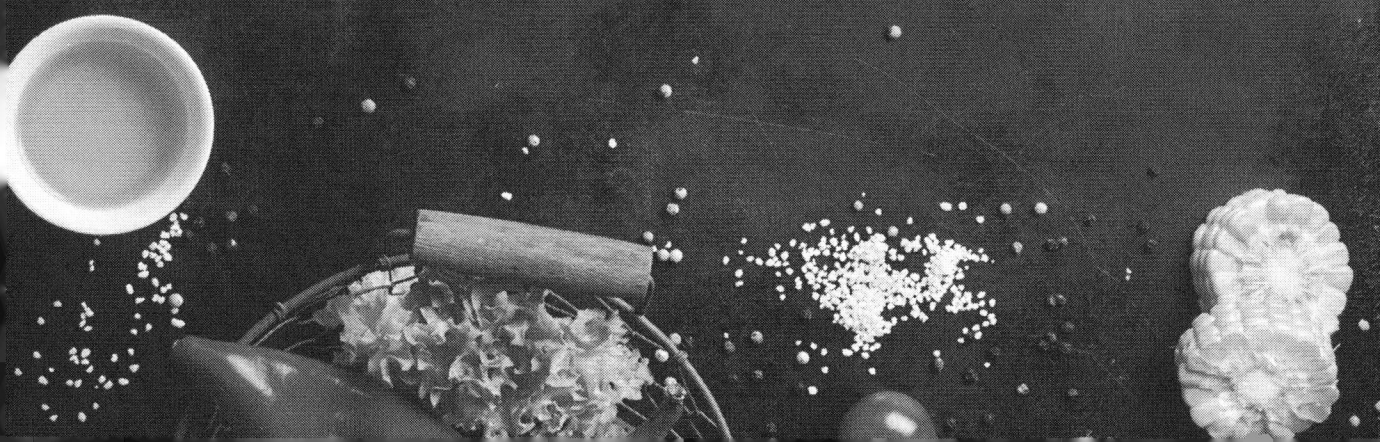

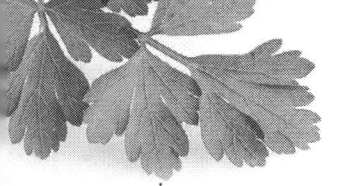

BBQ Bean and Chicken Bubble Up

(Prep Time: 10 MIN | Cook Time: 40 MIN | Serves: 6)

Ingredients:

For cooking:
Nonstick spray

For bubble up:
1 (15½ ounce) can navy beans (rinsed, drained)
12 ounces shredded cooked chicken breast
8 ounces canned tomato sauce
1 cup BBQ sauce
4 rashers centre-cut bacon (cooked, chopped)
1 (7½ ounce) can readymade biscuit dough (chilled)
4 ounces low-fat Cheddar cheese (shredded)

Directions:

1. Preheat the main oven to 350 degrees F. Spritz a 13x9" casserole dish with nonstick spray and set to one side.
2. Add the navy beans, shredded chicken, sauces, and cooked bacon to the casserole dish. Stir until well combined.
3. Break the biscuit dough into pieces and add to the casserole dish, gently stir to incorporate.
4. Place in the oven and bake for just under half an hour. Remove from the oven and scatter over the Cheddar. Pop back in the oven for 10-15 more minutes; the biscuits should have puffed up, and the cheese should have melted.
5. Slice into 6 portions and serve hot.

Freestyle Points Per Serving: 6

(Calories 375 | Total Fats 7g | Net Carbs: 41g | Protein 33g | Fiber: 4g)

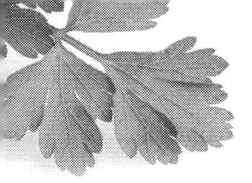

Coconut Breaded Chicken Tenders

(Prep Time: 15 MIN | Cook Time: 20 MIN | Serves: 4)

Ingredients:

For cooking:
Nonstick spray

For chicken:
Whites of 2 medium eggs (whisked)
1 pound chicken breast tenders

For coating:
1 tbsp turmeric
6 tbsp shredded coconut (unsweetened)
¼ tsp black pepper
½ tsp powdered garlic
Pinch red pepper flakes
¼ tsp kosher salt

Directions:

1. Preheat the main oven to 400 degrees F. Place a wire rack onto a baking tray and spritz with nonstick spray. Set to one side.
2. Add all coating ingredient to a shallow bowl and stir to combine.
3. In a second shallow bowl, add the egg whites.
4. Dip both sides of each chicken tender first in the egg white and then in the coating. Arrange on the wire rack.
5. Spritz the coated tenders with nonstick spray and place in the oven. Bake for 10-12 minutes before flipping and cooking for another several minutes.
6. Serve hot.

Freestyle Points Per Serving: 5

(Calories 2200 | Total Fats 6g | Net Carbs: 8g | Protein 30g | Fiber: 2g)

POULTRY

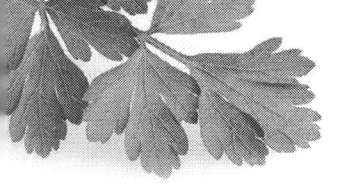

Cordon Bleu Skillet Chicken

(Prep Time: 15 MIN | Cook Time: 15 MIN | Serves: 4)

Ingredients:

For cooking:
1½ tsp olive oil
½ tsp salted butter

For chicken:
4 (4 ounce) skinless, boneless chicken cutlets
½ tsp sea salt
Pinch black pepper
¼ cup all-purpose flour
4 (¾ ounce slices) reduced-salt deli ham
4 (¾ ounce slices) low-fat Swiss cheese
Fresh parsley (chopped, for garnish)

For sauce:
⅔ cup fat-free chicken stock
1 tbsp freshly squeezed lemon juice
½ tbsp Dijon mustard
1 tsp all-purpose flour

Directions:

1. Season each chicken cutlet with sea salt and black pepper.
2. Add the flour to a wide dish. Dip each cutlet in the flour to coat both sides, shake off any excess and set aside for a moment.
3. Whisk together the sauce ingredients and set to one side.
4. Melt the oil and butter in a 12" skillet over moderately high heat. Add the floured chicken cutlets and sauté for 2 minutes on both sides. Transfer the semi-cooked chicken to a plate.
5. Add the set-aside sauce mixture to the skillet and scraping up any brown bits, bring the sauce to simmer for 2-3 minutes until it reduces a little.
6. Place the chicken back in the skillet and arrange one slice of ham and one slice of cheese on top of each piece.
7. Cover the skillet with a lid and cook at a moderately low simmer for 3-4 minutes until the cheese has melted.
8. Divide the chicken between four plates and spoon a little of the remaining sauce over each portion.

Freestyle Points Per Serving: 5

(Calories 260 | Total Fats 10g | Net Carbs 6g | Protein 37g | Fiber: 0g)

FREESTYLE 2018

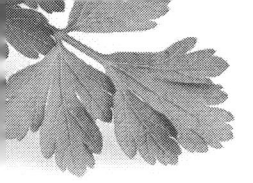

Feta and Butternut Squash Turkey Skillet

(Prep Time: 10 MIN | Cook Time: 20 MIN | Serves: 4)

Ingredients:

For cooking:
1 tbsp olive oil

Seasoning:
Sea salt and black pepper
1 tsp Italian seasoning mix
1 tsp powdered garlic
¼ tsp crushed red pepper flakes

For turkey:
1 pound 99% lean ground turkey
1 red bell pepper (seeded, diced)
½ yellow onion (peeled, minced)
2 cloves garlic (peeled, minced)
1 cup canned chopped tomatoes
2 cups butternut squash (peeled, seeded, chopped)
1 cup low-fat feta cheese (crumbled)

Directions:

1. To a large skillet, add the oil and place over moderately high heat. Add the turkey and sauté for several minutes; use a wooden spoon to break up the turkey as it cooks.
2. Add the red bell pepper, onion, and garlic, cook for another 5-6 minutes until the vegetables have softened.
3. Add the chopped tomatoes, chopped squash, and seasoning, stir well. Cover with a lid and cook for several minutes.
4. Add the feta cheese and recover for 2-3 minutes more until the cheese melts.
5. Serve.

Freestyle Points Per Serving: 3

(Calories 280 | Total Fats 10g | Net Carbs: 12g | Protein 35g | Fiber: 3g)

POULTRY

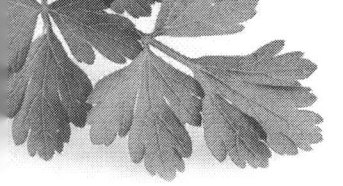

Honey and Balsamic Glazed Chicken

(Prep Time: 15 MIN | Cook Time: 20 MIN | Serves: 4)

Ingredients:

For cooking:
2 tsp olive oil

For chicken:
4 (6 ounce) skinless, boneless chicken breasts
2 tsp fresh thyme
½ tsp kosher salt
¼ tsp black pepper

For glaze:
2 tsp organic honey
¼ cup good quality balsamic vinegar
⅓ cup water
2 tbsp salted butter (chopped)

Directions:

1. Season the chicken breasts with thyme, kosher salt, and black pepper.
2. Add the oil to a skillet over moderate heat.
3. Place the chicken breasts in the skillet and cook for a few minutes on each side, until golden brown. Transfer to a side plate and tent with aluminum foil.
4. Add the honey, balsamic, and water to the same skillet and bring the mixture to a boil for 2-3 minutes, while continually stirring. Add the chopped butter and continue to cook until the butter has melted.
5. Turn the heat down to moderately low and pop the chicken breasts back in the skillet. Cook the chicken for a few more minutes on each side until cooked through.
6. Divide the chicken breasts between four serving plates and serve drizzled with remaining glaze.

Freestyle Points Per Serving: 5

(Calories 300 | Total Fats 6g | Net Carbs: 4g | Protein 38g | Fiber: 1g)

FREESTYLE 2018

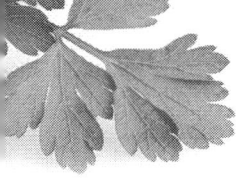

Moroccan Olive and Chicken Tagine

(Prep Time: 10 MIN | Cook Time: 6 HOUR | Serves: 4)

Ingredients:

For chicken:

8 skinless, boneless chicken thighs
⅓ cup dried prunes (sliced in half)
4 carrots (peeled, chopped)
½ cup green olives (pitted, chopped)
1 yellow onion (peeled, finely chopped)
1 cup reduced salt chicken stock
2 tbsp all-purpose flour

Seasoning:

2 tsp paprika
2 tsp cumin
1 tsp cinnamon
2 tsp fresh ginger (peeled, minced)
1 tsp salt
Pinch black pepper

Directions:

1. Add all of the chicken ingredients to a slow cooker (4-6 quart capacity) and stir well.
2. Add the seasoning and stir again, very well, until combined. Cover with a lid and cook for 6 hours on low heat.
3. Serve hot.

Freestyle Points Per Serving: 7

(Calories 400 | Total Fats 13g | Net Carbs: 19g | Protein 46g | Fiber: 5g)

POULTRY

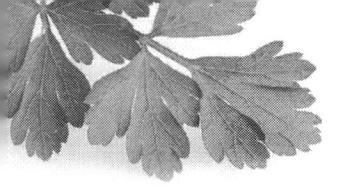

Rustic Leftover Turkey Broccoli Casserole

(Prep Time: 15 MIN | Cook Time: 30 MIN | Serves: 6)

Ingredients:

For cooking:
Nonstick spray

For casserole:
20 ounces leftover cooked broccoli (chopped)
3 skinless, boneless turkey breasts (cooked, chopped)
1 tsp freshly squeezed lemon juice
¾ cup non-fat evaporated milk
1 (22 ounce) can cream of chicken condensed soup (98% fat-free)
1 cup low-fat Cheddar cheese (shredded)
2 tbsp Parmesan cheese
½ cup seasoned breadcrumbs

Directions:

1. Preheat the main oven to 350 degrees F. Spritz a 13x9" casserole dish with nonstick spray and set to one side.
2. Add the chopped broccoli and turkey to a large bowl and toss to combine.
3. In a second bowl, add the lemon juice, milk, and chicken soup. Stir well to combine and then pour over the turkey and broccoli. Toss until the turkey and broccoli are well coated and transfer to the casserole dish.
4. Scatter over the Cheddar cheese.
5. In a small bowl, combine the Parmesan and breadcrumbs and then sprinkle over the Cheddar.
6. Spritz the top of the casserole with nonstick spray and place in the oven. Bake for just under half an hour until bubbling.
7. Allow to cool for a few minutes before serving.

Freestyle Points Per Serving: 7

(Calories 360 | Total Fats 14g | Net Carbs: 20g | Protein 37g | Fiber: 4g)

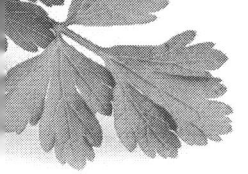

Shepherd's Pie with Sweet Potato

(Prep Time: 15 MIN | Cook Time: 1 HOUR | Serves: 6)

Ingredients:

For cooking:

1 tsp olive oil

For sweet potato topping:

3 garlic cloves (peeled)
1½ pounds sweet potato (peeled, finely chopped)
¼ cup fat-free chicken stock
½ cup skim milk
Sea salt and black pepper
2 tbsp low-fat sour cream

For turkey filling:

1 pound 95% lean ground turkey
Sea salt and black pepper
1 yellow onion (peeled, finely chopped)
1 medium parsnip (peeled, chopped)
1 stalk celery (chopped)
8 ounces fresh mushrooms (finely chopped)
2 garlic cloves (peeled, finely chopped)
2 tbsp flour
2 tsp tomato paste
1 cup fat-free chicken stock
10 ounces mixed vegetables (frozen)
1 tsp Worcestershire sauce
1 tsp fresh rosemary (chopped)
Pinch paprika

Directions:

1. In a deep pot of salted, boiling water cook the garlic and chopped potatoes. When soft and fully cooked, drain away the water and add the remaining potato topping ingredients to the pot. Mash well until totally combined and relatively smooth. Set to one side.
2. Preheat the main oven to 400 degrees F.
3. In a skillet over moderate heat, sauté the ground turkey and season well. When browned and fully cooked, set to one side.
4. Using the same skillet, sauté the onion in the olive oil for 60 seconds then add the parsnip and celery. Season again and cook for 10-12 minutes until the vegetables are soft.
5. Add the mushrooms and garlic cooking for another few minutes.
6. Sprinkle in the flour and stir well before adding the tomato paste, chicken stock, mixed vegetables, Worcestershire sauce, set-aside turkey, rosemary, and paprika. Cook at a simmer for several minutes.
7. Divide the meat mixture between 6 small oven-safe dishes. Top each portion with half a cup of the prepared sweet potato mash, spreading out into an even layer.
8. Place in the oven and bake for 20-25 minutes, allow to cool for several minutes before serving.

Freestyle Points Per Serving: 8

(Calories 250 | Total Fats 6g | Net Carbs: 28g | Protein 16.5g | Fiber: 6g)

POULTRY

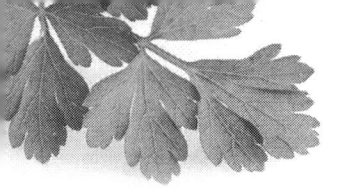

Slow Cooked Chicken with Mushrooms

(Prep Time: 10 MIN | Cook Time: 8 HOUR | Serves: 8)

Ingredients:

For chicken:

5 pounds skinless, boneless chicken breasts
Sea salt and black pepper
1 yellow onion (peeled, chopped)
8 ounces mushrooms (thickly sliced)
1 (24 ounce) can tomato soup

For vegetables:

2 small zucchini (sliced)
12 ounces fresh broccoli (chopped into florets)

Directions:

1. Add all of the chicken ingredients to a slow cooker and stir well until combined. Cover with a lid and cook for 7 hours on low heat.
2. Remove the chicken breasts and check to see that they are cooked through. Shred with two forks. Return to the slow cooker along with the zucchini and broccoli.
3. Re-cover and cook for another hour before serving.

Freestyle Points Per Serving: 2

(Calories 345 | Total Fats 6g | Net Carbs: 17g | Protein 55g | Fiber: 2g)

FREESTYLE 2018

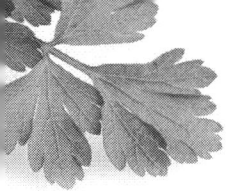

Sweet and Smoky Apricot Chicken

(Prep Time: 50 MIN | Cook Time: 30 MIN | Serves: 6)

Ingredients:

For chicken:
1 pound skinless, boneless chicken breasts

For sauce:
½ cup sugar-free smoky BBQ sauce
½ cup sugar-free apricot jam
1 tsp powdered garlic
2 tbsp soy sauce
1 tsp powdered ginger
1 tsp onion powder

Directions:

1. Preheat the main oven to 350 degrees F. Cover a baking tray with aluminum foil.
2. Arrange the chicken breasts on the baking tray in an even layer.
3. Whisk together all of the sauce ingredients in a small bowl. Pour the sauce evenly over the breasts.
4. Place in the oven and cook for half an hour, until cooked through.
5. Enjoy.

Freestyle Points Per Serving: 2

(Calories 215 | Total Fats 5.5g | Net Carbs: 15.5g | Protein 23g | Fiber: 0.5g)

POULTRY

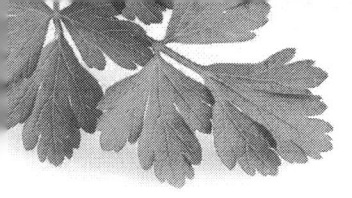

Thai Spiced Peanut Chicken

 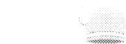

(Prep Time: 10 MIN | Cook Time: 5 HOUR 40 MIN | Serves: 9)

Ingredients:

For peanut chicken:

2 pounds skinless, boneless chicken breasts
½ cup low-calorie orange juice
¾ cup peanut butter powder mixed with 6 tbsp water
¼ cup reduced-calorie orange marmalade
2 tbsp soy sauce
1½ tbsp sesame oil
2 tbsp hoisin sauce
2 tbsp teriyaki sauce
¼ tsp red pepper flakes (crushed)
¾ cup light canned coconut milk
1 clove garlic (peeled, minced)

Directions:

1. Add all of the ingredients to a slow cooker, stir very well until combined.
2. Cover with a lid and cook on low heat for 5 ½ hours, until the chicken is completely cooked.
3. Transfer the chicken breasts to a plate and shred using two metal forks. Return the shredded chicken to the slow cooker and stir thoroughly. Cook for several more minutes before serving.

Freestyle Points Per Serving: 3

(Calories 205 | Total Fats 6g | Net Carbs: 11g | Protein 27g | Fiber: 1g)

Red Meat

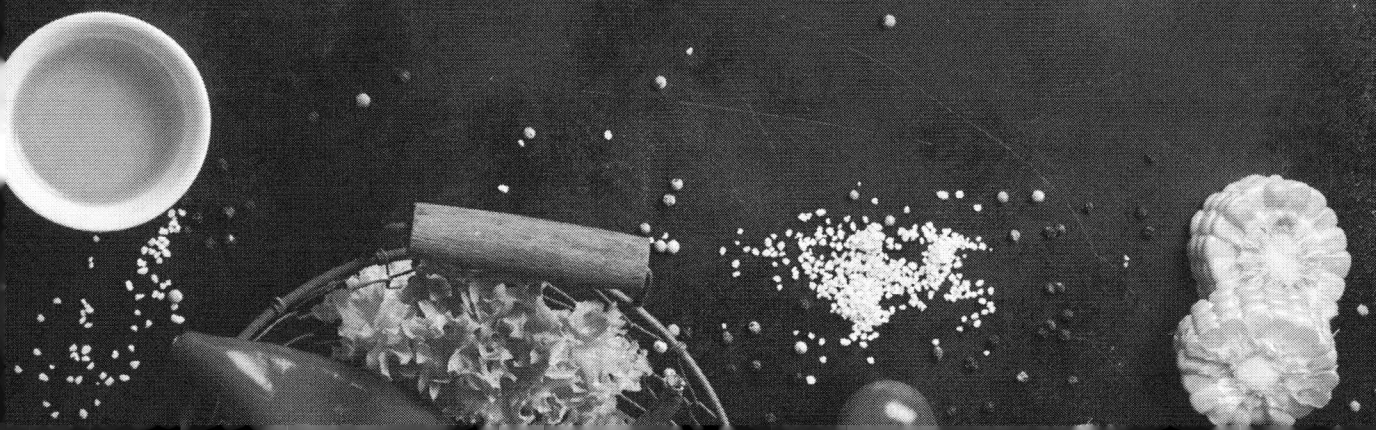

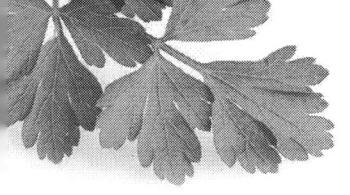

African Harissa Grilled Lamb

(Prep Time: 8 HOUR 10 MIN | Cook Time: 10 MIN | Serves: 4)

Ingredients:

For cooking:

Nonstick spray

For lamb:

8 (3½ ounce) lamb loin bone-in chops
4 garlic cloves (peeled, crushed)
2 tbsp freshly squeezed lemon juice
2 tbsp Harissa paste
Sea salt and black pepper
¾ tsp cumin

Directions:

1. Add all of the lamb ingredients to a large dish mixing well with hands until the lamb is covered well with the other ingredients. Cover and chill overnight.
2. When ready to cook, spritz a grill pan with nonstick spray and place over moderately high heat.
3. Cook the chops for 5 minutes on each side, until medium-rare and enjoy straight away.

Freestyle Points Per Serving: 5

(Calories 200 | Total Fats 8g | Net Carbs: 1g | Protein 30g | Fiber: 1g)

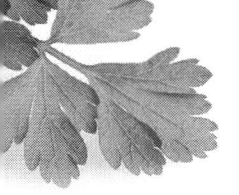

Bacon Burger Quesadillas

(Prep Time: 15 MIN | Cook Time: 20 MIN | Serves: 5)

Ingredients:

For cooking:

Nonstick spray

For quesadillas:

½ cup yellow onion (peeled, diced)

1 pound ground beef 95% lean

1 tbsp hamburger seasoning

3 rashers centre-cut bacon (cooked until crispy, crumbled)

4 tbsp low-carb BBQ sauce

10 low-calorie yellow corn tortillas

5 ounces low-fat Cheddar cheese (grated)

Directions:

1. Spritz a skillet with nonstick spray and place over moderate heat.
2. Add the onion and sauté for 3-4 minutes until soft.
3. Add the beef and sauté until cooked through. Use a wooden spoon to try to break up the meat as it cooks.
4. Drain away any excess fat from the pan and sprinkle in the burger seasoning, stirring well to coat the meat.
5. Add the crumbled bacon and BBQ sauce, stir well and then take off the heat. Set aside for a moment.
6. Take five of the tortillas and spritz them on one side with nonstick spray.
7. Arrange the tortillas, sprayed side down, on a large griddle pan. Onto each tortilla, sprinkle half an ounce of grated Cheddar and spoon half a cup of the beef mixture. Use the back of a spoon to gently spread the beef mixture into an even layer.
8. Take the remaining five tortillas and again, spritz only one side with nonstick spray. Use these tortillas to top the tortillas in the griddle pan (spritzed side facing up).
9. Place the griddle pan over moderately high heat for approximately 4 minutes, until the cheese is melting. Use a spatula to flip each quesadilla, cook for another few minutes before slicing each quesadilla into quarters and serving hot.

Freestyle Points Per Serving: 8

(Calories 300 | Total Fats 11g | Net Carbs: 27g | Protein 31g | Fiber: 3g)

RED MEAT

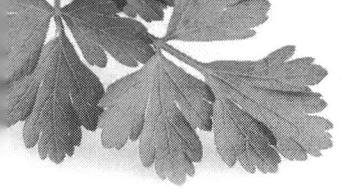

Cornflake Crusted Pork Chops

(Prep Time: 10 MIN | Cook Time: 20 MIN | Serves: 6)

Ingredients:

For cooking:
Nonstick spray

For pork:
½ tsp kosher salt
6 (5 ounce) centre-cut pork chops (trimmed of fat)
1 egg (beaten)

For crust:
½ cup panko breadcrumbs
⅓ cup cornflakes (crushed)
2 tbsp Parmesan cheese (finely grated)
½ tsp powdered garlic
1¼ tsp paprika
¾ tsp kosher salt
¼ tsp chili powder
½ tsp onion powder
Pinch black pepper

Directions:

1. Preheat an air fryer to 400 degrees F and spritz the metal basket with nonstick spray.
2. Sprinkle salt on both sides of each pork chop. Set aside for a moment.
3. Add the beaten egg to a bowl. Add all of the crust ingredients to a second bowl and stir to combine.
4. Working in two batches of three chops, dip each pork chop first in the egg and then in the crust.
5. Place in the air fryer and spritz with more nonstick spray. Cook for 6 minutes on each side.
6. Repeat with the remaining chops and serve.

Freestyle Points Per Serving: 7

(Calories 375 | Total Fats 13g | Net Carbs: 8g | Protein 33g | Fiber: 0g)

FREESTYLE 2018

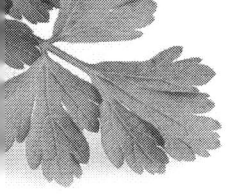

Hearty Beef and Barley Casserole

(Prep Time: 10 MIN | Cook Time: 4 HOUR | Serves: 8)

Ingredients:

For casserole:

2 pounds lean, boneless, trimmed beef chuck steak (cut into small chunks)
1 cup canned tomato sauce
2 stalks celery (finely chopped)
1 yellow onion (peeled, chopped)
5 carrots (thinly sliced)
6 cups fat-free beef stock
1 cup mushrooms (sliced)
1 tsp black pepper
3 cloves garlic (peeled, minced)
¼ cup fresh parsley (chopped)
1 cup pearl barley
2 tbsp Worcestershire sauce
2 tsp kosher salt

Directions:

1. Add all of the ingredients to a slow cooker, stir very well until combined.
2. Cook for 4 hours on high heat and serve hot.

Freestyle Points Per Serving: 6

(Calories 275 | Total Fats 6g | Net Carbs: 23g | Protein 28g | Fiber: 5g)

RED MEAT

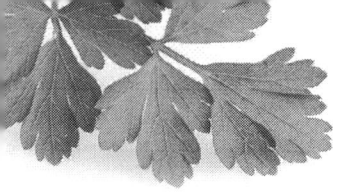

Korean Beef Bowls

(Prep Time: 10 MIN | Cook Time: 15 MIN | Serves: 4)

Ingredients:

For beef:
2 tbsp water
3 cups mixed Asian vegetables
1⅓ pounds 97% lean ground beef

For sauce:
¼ cup soy sauce
2 tbsp light brown sugar
2 tsp sesame oil
1 tsp Asian chili paste with garlic
2 cloves garlic (peeled, minced)
1 tbsp fresh ginger (peeled, minced)

Directions:

1. Add the water and mixed vegetables to a pan over moderately high heat, cook for a few minutes until crispy yet tender. Set to one side.
2. Using the same pan, cook the beef until brown and cooked through. Use a wooden spoon to break up the meat as it cooks.
3. While the meat cooks, whisk together all of the sauce ingredients and add to the pan. Bring to a simmer for 4-5 minutes.
4. Return the vegetables to the skillet and stir well to combine.
5. Serve.

Freestyle Points Per Serving: 6

(Calories 295 | Total Fats 10g | Net Carbs: 14g | Protein 35g | Fiber: 3g)

FREESTYLE 2018

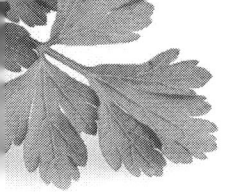

Peach and Ginger Roast Pork Tenderloin

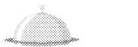

(Prep Time: 15 MIN | Cook Time: 30 MIN | Serves: 4)

Ingredients:

For cooking:
2 tsp canola oil

For pork:
1 (1 pound) pork tenderloin (fat trimmed)
Sea salt and black pepper
¼ cup dry white wine

For sauce:
1 (14½ ounce) can no added sugar sliced peaches (rinsed, drained)
2 tsp fresh ginger (peeled, grated)
1 tbsp soy sauce
1 cloves garlic (peeled, minced)
½ tsp hot sauce

Directions:

1. Preheat the main oven to 425 degrees F. Cover a baking tray with foil and set to one side.
2. Add all of the sauce ingredients to a blender and blitz until smooth. Set to one side.
3. Season the tenderloin with sea salt and black pepper.
4. Add the oil to a skillet and place over moderately high heat. Add the pork to the skillet and cook for 4 minutes on each side, to seal in its juices. Transfer the pork to the baking tray.
5. Brush the tenderloin with 2 tbsp of the prepared sauce. Place in the oven and roast for just under 20 minutes until cooked through.
6. Add the remaining sauce to a saucepan over moderately high heat along with the dry white wine. Bring to a boil then turn down to a simmer for 10 minutes.
7. Slice the pork and divide between four serving plates serve with the peach/wine sauce.

Freestyle Points Per Serving: 6

(Calories 197 | Total Fats 6g | Net Carbs: 6g | Protein 24g | Fiber: 1g)

RED MEAT

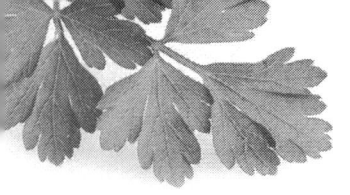

Philly Cheesesteak Mushrooms

(Prep Time: 15 MIN | Cook Time: 30 MIN | Serves: 4)

Ingredients:

For cooking:
Nonstick spray

For cheese sauce:
¼ cup low-fat sour cream
2 tbsp low-fat mayo
2 ounces low-fat cream cheese (at room temperature)
3 ounces low-fat Cheddar cheese (shredded)

For steak mushrooms:
4 Portobello mushrooms
Sea salt and black pepper
6 ounces sirloin steak (sliced into thin strips)
¾ cup green bell pepper (seeded, diced)
¾ cup yellow onion (peeled, diced)

Directions:

1. Preheat the main oven to 400 degrees F. Spritz a baking tray with nonstick spray.
2. First, prepare the mushrooms. Remove their stems and gills then spritz with nonstick spray and season with sea salt and black pepper. Set to one side.
3. Season the steak strips with sea salt and black pepper.
4. Spritz a skillet with nonstick spray and place over high heat. Add the steak to the skillet and sauté for 60-90 seconds on each side until cooked. Transfer to a plate.
5. Spritz the same skillet with more nonstick spray and place over moderately low heat.
6. Add the bell pepper and onion to the skillet and sauté for 5 minutes until soft. Take off the heat and set to one side.
7. Add all of the cheese sauce ingredients to a medium bowl and stir until well combined. Add the strips of steak, cooked peppers, and onion to the cheese mixture.
8. Arrange the mushroom caps on the baking tray and stuff each with half a cup of the cheesesteak mixture.
9. Place in the oven and bake for 20 minutes until the cheesesteak mixture is melted and bubbling.
10. Serve hot.

Freestyle Points Per Serving: 7

(Calories 255 | Total Fats 16g | Net Carbs: 6g | Protein 20g | Fiber: 4g)

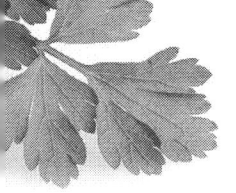

Spicy Pepper Cubed Steak

(Prep Time: 10 MIN | Cook Time: 25 MIN | Serves: 8)

Ingredients:

For cubed steak:

28 ounces cubed steak
Pinch black pepper
1¾ tsp garlic salt
1 red bell pepper (seeded, sliced)
½ red onion (peeled, sliced)
1 cup water
8 ounces canned tomato sauce
2 tbsp brine (from olive jar)
⅓ cup green olives (pitted)

Directions:

1. Season the cubed steak with black pepper and garlic salt, add to a pressure cooker along with the bell pepper and onion.
2. Pour over the water, tomato sauce, and brine, stir well until combined then fold in the olives.
3. Cover with a lid and cook for 25 minutes on a high setting.
4. Serve.

Freestyle Points Per Serving: 2

(Calories 155 | Total Fats 5.5g | Net Carbs: 3g | Protein 23.5g | Fiber: 1g)

RED MEAT

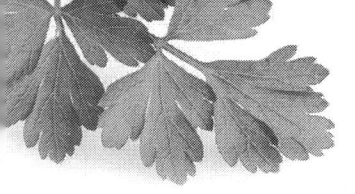

Swedish Meatballs in Creamy Gravy

(Prep Time: 15 MIN | Cook Time: 30 MIN | Serves: 4)

Ingredients:

For cooking:
1 tsp olive oil

For gravy:
2 cups fat-free beef stock
2 ounces low-fat cream cheese

For meatballs:
1 garlic cloves (peeled, minced)
1 yellow onion (peeled, minced)
¼ cup fresh parsley (minced)
1 stalk celery (minced)
1 pound ground beef 95% lean
Kosher salt and black pepper
¼ cup seasoned breadcrumbs
1 egg
½ tsp allspice

Directions:

1. Add the oil to a frying pan and place over moderate heat.
2. Add the garlic and onion to the pan, sauté for 4 minutes until soft.
3. Add the parsley and celery, sauté for another 3 minutes. Transfer to a mixing bowl and set aside until cool enough to handle.
4. Add the remaining meatball ingredients to the mixing bowl and combine using clean hands.
5. Roll the mixture into equally-sized balls.
6. Using the same frying pan as before, bring the beef stock to a boil over moderately high heat. Turn the heat down to moderately low and add the meatballs to the pan.
7. Cover with a lid and cook for 20 minutes. Remove the cooked meatballs from the broth using a slotted spoon and set to one side.
8. Transfer the stock to a blender along with the cream cheese and blitz until smooth. Pour the creamy gravy back into the pan and bring to a simmer for 3-4 minutes.
9. Divide the meatballs equally between serving plates and serve with the creamy gravy.

Freestyle Points Per Serving: 6

(Calories 215 | Total Fats 10g | Net Carbs: 8g | Protein 25g | Fiber: 1g)

FREESTYLE 2018

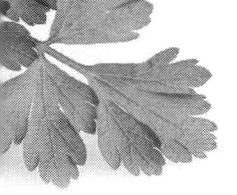

Sweet Mustard Spiral Ham

(Prep Time: 10 MIN | Cook Time: 5 HOUR 30 MIN | Serves: 16)

Ingredients:

For glaze:

2 tbsp Dijon mustard
5 tbsp apricot preserves

For ham:

1 (6½ pound) Hickory smoked spiral-cut ham (fully cooked)
1 tbsp apricot preserves

Directions:

1. Whisk together the glaze ingredients and set to one side for a moment.
2. Arrange the cooked ham in a large slow cooker and brush with the glaze. Cover with a lid and cook for 4-5 hours on a low setting.
3. Remove the lid and brush with 1 tbsp apricot preserves, re-cover and cook for a final half an hour.
4. Slice and serve!

Freestyle Points Per Serving: 5

(Calories 145 | Total Fats 7g | Net Carbs: 12g | Protein 15g | Fiber: 0g)

RED MEAT

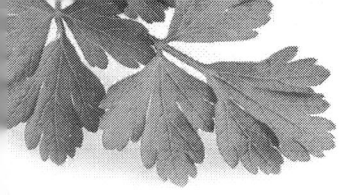

Zesty Lime and Garlic Pork Chops

(Prep Time: 35 MIN | Cook Time: 10 MIN | Serves: 4)

Ingredients:

For marinade:

4 garlic cloves (peeled, crushed)
1 tsp lime zest (grated)
½ tsp sweet paprika
½ tsp cumin
Juice of ½ a medium lime
½ tsp chili powder

For pork:

4 boneless, lean pork chops (fat trimmed)
Sea salt and black pepper

Directions:

1. Add all of the marinade ingredients to a shallow dish and stir well to combine.
2. Season the pork chops on both sides with sea salt and black pepper and then arrange them in the marinade. Chill for half an hour.
3. To cook the chops, grill on moderately high heat for 5 minutes on both sides. Enjoy hot.

Freestyle Points Per Serving: 5

(Calories 225 | Total Fats 6g | Net Carbs: 2g | Protein 38g | Fiber: 0g)

Seafood

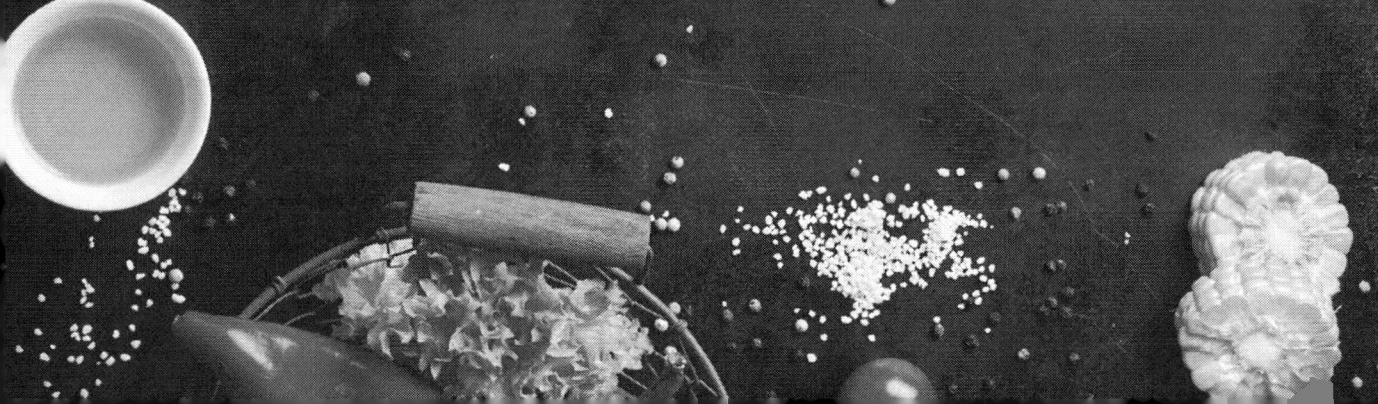

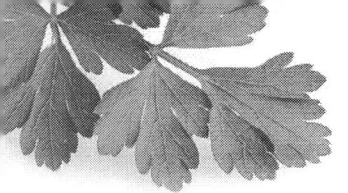

Blackened Halibut Tacos with Fruity Slaw

(Prep Time: 10 MIN | Cook Time: 10 MIN | Serves: 4)

Ingredients:

For cooking:
Nonstick spray

For fruity slaw:
3½ cups red cabbage (finely shredded)
Juice of 1 medium lime
1 ripe mango
(peeled, pitted, sliced into matchsticks)
½ tsp sea salt
2 tsp olive oil
¼ cup fresh cilantro (chopped)

For blackened seasoning:
½ tsp cayenne pepper
½ tsp mustard powder
1 tsp paprika
¼ tsp cumin
1 tsp salt
Pinch black pepper
¼ tsp oregano

For tacos:
½ medium lime
1 pound skinless halibut fillets
8 corn tortillas (warmed)

Directions:

1. Add all slaw ingredients to a bowl and toss until well combined. Keep chilled until ready to serve.
2. Combine all of the seasoning ingredients in a small bowl.
3. Take the lime half and squeeze it over the halibut, then rub the fish with the seasoning until well coated.
4. Place a skillet over high heat and spritz with nonstick spray. Add the fish and cook for 5 minutes on both sides until cooked through. Transfer to a plate.
5. Break the fish into large chunks and divide between the warm tortillas. Top each with half a cup of prepared slaw and serve straight away.

Freestyle Points Per Serving: 4

(Calories 275 | Total Fats 5g | Net Carbs: 26g | Protein 30g | Fiber: 5g)

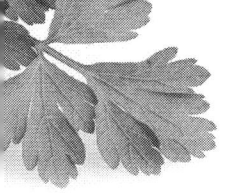

Chickpea, Caper, and Tuna Salad

(Prep Time: 5 MIN | Cook Time: N/A | Serves: 2)

Ingredients:

For tuna salad:
1 (6 ounce) can tuna in water (drained)
1 (15 ounce) can chickpeas (drained, rinsed)
2 tbsp red wine vinegar
2 tbsp capers in brine + 2 tbsp brine
1½ tbsp red onion (finely chopped)

For serving:
Iceberg lettuce (shredded)

Directions:

1. Add all of the tuna salad ingredients to a medium-sized bowl and mix until well combined.
2. Serve the tuna salad over shredded iceberg lettuce.

Freestyle Points Per Serving: 0

(Calories 275 | Total Fats 3g | Net Carbs: 28g | Protein 27g | Fiber: 8g)

SEAFOOD

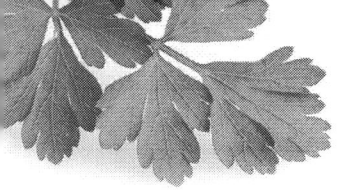

Crispy Shrimp Taquitos

(Prep Time: 15 MIN | Cook Time: 30 MIN | Serves: 6)

Ingredients:

For cooking:
Nonstick spray
1 tsp olive oil

For taquitos:
1 jalapeno (seeded, minced)
2 garlic cloves (peeled, minced)
½ yellow onion (peeled, diced)
1 tomato (diced)
12 ounces fresh shrimp (peeled, deveined, chopped)
2 tbsp fresh cilantro (finely chopped)
¼ tsp sea salt
12 low-calorie yellow corn tortillas
¾ cup pepper jack cheese (shredded)

Directions:

1. Preheat the main oven to 400 degrees F and cover two baking sheets with aluminum foil. Spritz the foil with nonstick spray.
2. Add the olive oil to a skillet and place over moderate heat.
3. Add the jalapeno, garlic, and onion, sauté for 3-4 minutes until soft.
4. Add the diced tomato and sauté for another few minutes before adding the chopped shrimp, cilantro, and sea salt. Increase the heat to moderately high and sauté for 60 seconds. Take off the heat.
5. Working in batches of four, microwave the tortillas for 30 seconds until soft and warm.
6. Spoon 3 tbsp of filling onto each tortilla and sprinkle with 1 tbsp shredded cheese. Roll up each tortilla like a burrito and arrange on the baking sheets, seam side down.
7. Spritz the taquitos with nonstick spray and place in the oven. Bake for 15 minutes until the tortillas are crispy and golden.

Freestyle Points Per Serving: 5

(Calories 245 | Total Fats 8g | Net Carbs: 24g | Protein 18g | Fiber: 4g)

FREESTYLE 2018

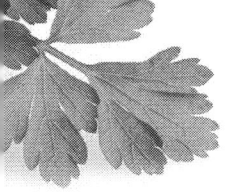

Garlic and Herb Tilapia

(Prep Time: 10 MIN | Cook Time: 8 MIN | Serves: 6)

Ingredients:

For herb and garlic seasoning:

3 tsp olive oil
2 garlic cloves (peeled, crushed)
1 tsp parsley
1 tsp oregano
Kosher salt and black pepper

For fish:

6 (6 ounce) fresh tilapia fillets
2 lemon halves

Directions:

1. Preheat your broiler to a low heat setting.
2. Add all of the seasoning ingredients to a small bowl and stir to combine.
3. Arrange aluminum foil inside a broiler pan and set the tilapia on top. Drizzle the fish evenly with the seasoning and squeeze over the two lemon halves.
4. Arrange the pan several inches away from the flame and cook for 7-8 minutes until cooked through. Serve straight away.

Freestyle Points Per Serving: 1

(Calories 200 | Total Fats 6.5g | Net Carbs: 1.5g | Protein 35g | Fiber: 1g)

SEAFOOD

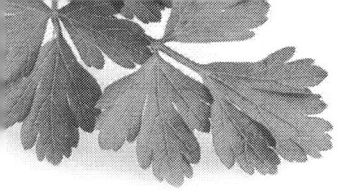

Grilled Lemon and Salmon Kebabs

(Prep Time: 10 MIN | Cook Time: 10 MIN | Serves: 4)

Ingredients:

For cooking:
Nonstick spray

Seasoning:
2 tbsp fresh oregano (finely chopped)
2 tsp sesame seeds
1 tsp cumin
¼ tsp red pepper flakes (crushed)
1 tsp sea salt

For kebabs:
1½ pounds salmon fillet (skin removed, chopped into 1" chunks)
2 lemons (sliced)
8 metal kebab skewers

Directions:

1. Preheat a grill to moderately high heat and spritz the grates with nonstick spray.
2. Add the seasoning to a small bowl and stir to combine. Set to one side.
3. Thread the salmon chunks and lemon slices equally onto the kebab skewers, making sure to begin and end with salmon. Folding the lemon slices in half before skewering.
4. Spritz the kebabs with nonstick spray and sprinkle generously with the seasoning mixture.
5. To cook; grill the fish for 8-9 minutes, turning a few times, on the preheated grill. Enjoy hot.

Freestyle Points Per Serving: 0

(Calories 265 | Total Fats 10g | Net Carbs: 4g | Protein 35g | Fiber: 3g)

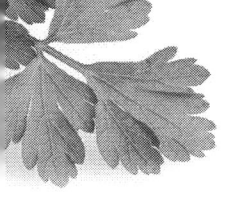

Hot Crab Salad Stuffed Avocado

(Prep Time: 10 MIN | Cook Time: N/A | Serves: 2)

Ingredients:

For crab salad:

2 tsp Asian hot sauce
2 tbsp low-fat mayo
1 tsp fresh chives (chopped)
4 ounces lump crabmeat
¼ cup cucumber (peeled, diced)

For avocado:

1 small, ripe avocado (halved lengthwise, pitted)
½ tsp sesame seeds
2 tsp soy sauce

Directions:

1. Add all of the crab salad ingredients to a small bowl and stir gently but well until combined.
2. Spoon the crab salad into the avocado halves. Sprinkle with sesame seeds and drizzle with soy. Serve straight away.

Freestyle Points Per Serving: 5

(Calories 195 | Total Fats 13g | Net Carbs: 3g | Protein 12g | Fiber: 4g)

SEAFOOD

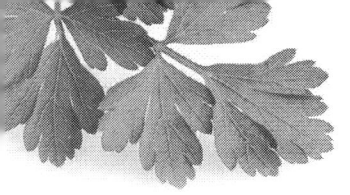

Lobster Salad with Asparagus

(Prep Time: 10 MIN | Cook Time: 3 MIN | Serves: 2)

Ingredients:

For dressing:
- 4 tsp virgin olive oil
- 2 tbsp freshly squeezed lemon juice
- ¼ tsp sea salt
- Pinch black pepper

For salad:
- 3½ cups fresh asparagus (chopped)
- 8 ounces fresh lobster (cooked, chopped)
- ½ cup cherry tomatoes (chopped)
- 2 tbsp red onion (diced)
- 3-4 fresh basil leaves

Directions:

1. Combine the dressing ingredients in a small bowl and set to one side.
2. In a medium-sized pot of boiling water, cook the chopped asparagus for a few minutes. Drain and set aside to cool.
3. Transfer the cooked asparagus to a serving bowl along with all of the remaining salad ingredients. Toss to combine.
4. Pour over the set-aside dressing and toss again until well coated.
5. Divide the salad between two plates and serve.

Freestyle Points Per Serving: 3

(Calories 250 | Total Fats 11g | Net Carbs: 9g | Protein 27g | Fiber: 5g)

FREESTYLE 2018

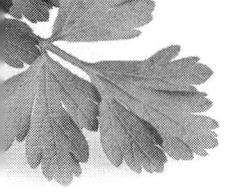

Mussels in White Wine and Basil Cream

(Prep Time: 10 MIN | Cook Time: 20 MIN | Serves: 3)

Ingredients:

For cooking:
2 tsp salted butter

For mussels:
1 garlic clove (peeled, finely chopped)
1 shallot (minced)
½ cup dry white wine
2 pounds fresh mussels (scrubbed, debearded, unopened mussels discarded)
¼ cup fat-free half & half

For sauce:
¼ cup fat-free half & half
2 garlic cloves (peeled, smashed)
2 tbsp olive oil
¼ cup Parmesan cheese (grated)
½ cup fresh basil leaves
Sea salt and black pepper

Directions:

1. First, prepare the mussels. In a deep saucepan, melt the butter. Add the garlic and shallot, sauté for 3-4 minutes. Pour in the wine and heat until boiling.
2. Add the mussels and cook, covered, for approximately 5 minutes until the mussels 'pop' open.
3. Transfer the cooked mussels to a serving bowl leaving the sauce behind in the pan. Discard any mussels that have not properly opened.
4. Add the half & half to the pan and bring to a simmer for 4-5 minutes.
5. In the meantime, add all of the sauce ingredients to a blender and blitz until pureed, add to the pan.
6. Stir the sauce in the pan well, while cooking for another 3-4 minutes. When hot-through, pour over the cooked mussels and serve straight away.

Freestyle Points Per Serving: 7

(Calories 370 | Total Fats 24g | Net Carbs: 11.5g | Protein 20.5g | Fiber: 0.5g)

SEAFOOD

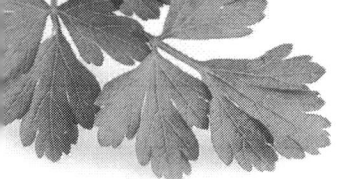

Seared Scallop Tostadas with Homemade Guacamole

(Prep Time: 15 MIN | Cook Time: 3 MIN | Serves: 2)

Ingredients:

For cooking:
1 tsp olive oil
1 tsp butter

For scallop tostadas:
8 ounces fresh scallops
Pinch black pepper
¼ tsp sea salt
2 corn tostada shells
2 tbsp low-fat sour cream mixed with 1 tsp fat-free milk

For guacamole:
¼ cup tomato (diced)
1 (4 ounce) ripe avocado (peeled, pitted, mashed)
2 tsp fresh cilantro (roughly chopped)
2 tbsp red onion (diced)
2 tsp freshly squeezed lime juice
Pinch black pepper
½ tsp sea salt

Directions:

1. Add all of the guacamole ingredients to a small bowl and stir until well combined. Set to one side.
2. Season the scallops on both sides with pepper and sea salt.
3. In a large skillet, melt the olive oil and butter over high heat. Sauté the scallops for 90 seconds on each side.
4. Divide the scallops between the tostada shells, drizzle with the milk/sour cream and top with guacamole. Serve straight away.

Freestyle Points Per Serving: 7

(Calories 295 | Total Fats 18g | Net Carbs: 15g | Protein 17g | Fiber: 5g)

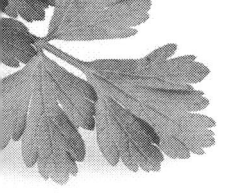

Swordfish Steak Burgers

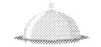

(Prep Time: 15 MIN | Cook Time: 10 MIN | Serves: 4)

Ingredients:

For cooking:
Nonstick spray

For lemon drizzle:
Juice of 1 medium lemon
8 tsp olive oil
Sea salt and black pepper

For burgers:
1½ pounds fresh, skinless swordfish steaks (chopped into chunks)
1 shallot
2 cloves garlic (peeled, chopped)
3 tbsp fresh chives (chopped)
Sea salt and black pepper
¼ cup breadcrumbs
2 tsp lemon zest (grated)
Romaine lettuce (chopped)

Directions:

1. Combine all of the lemon drizzle ingredients in a small bowl and set to one side.
2. Transfer a quarter of the swordfish chunks to a food processor. Set the remaining fish aside for a moment.
3. To the food processor, also add the shallot, garlic, and chives. Pulse until you have a thick paste. Transfer to a bowl.
4. Add the set-aside swordfish chunks to the food processor, pulse until chopped finely. Transfer to the bowl with the swordfish paste along with the sea salt and black pepper, breadcrumbs, and lemon zest. Combine using hands.
5. Shape the mixture into four burger patties.
6. To cook the burgers; spritz a skillet with nonstick spray and place over moderately high heat.
7. Cook the patties for 4-5 minutes each side.
8. Serve on a bed of romaine lettuce and drizzle with the lemon dressing.

Freestyle Points Per Serving: 4

(Calories 305 | Total Fats 16g | Net Carbs: 4g | Protein 33g | Fiber: 1g)

SEAFOOD

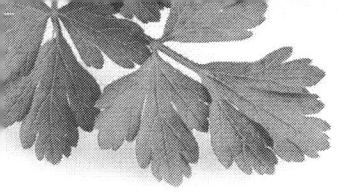

Zucchini Wrapped Cod

(Prep Time: 10 MIN | Cook Time: 10 MIN | Serves: 4)

Ingredients:

For cooking:

½ tbsp olive oil

For cod:

24 ounces skinless cod fillets

1 tbsp blackening seasoning

2 medium zucchinis (sliced into long strips)

Directions:

1. Season the cod fillets using half of the blackening seasoning.
2. Use the zucchini strips to wrap each fillet of cod and sprinkle with the remaining seasoning.
3. Add the oil to a large skillet and place the fillets inside, seam side down.
4. Cook for a few minutes on each side until white-through. Serve straight away.

Freestyle Points Per Serving: 1

(Calories 185 | Total Fats 3g | Net Carbs: 3g | Protein 37g | Fiber: 2g)

Snacks

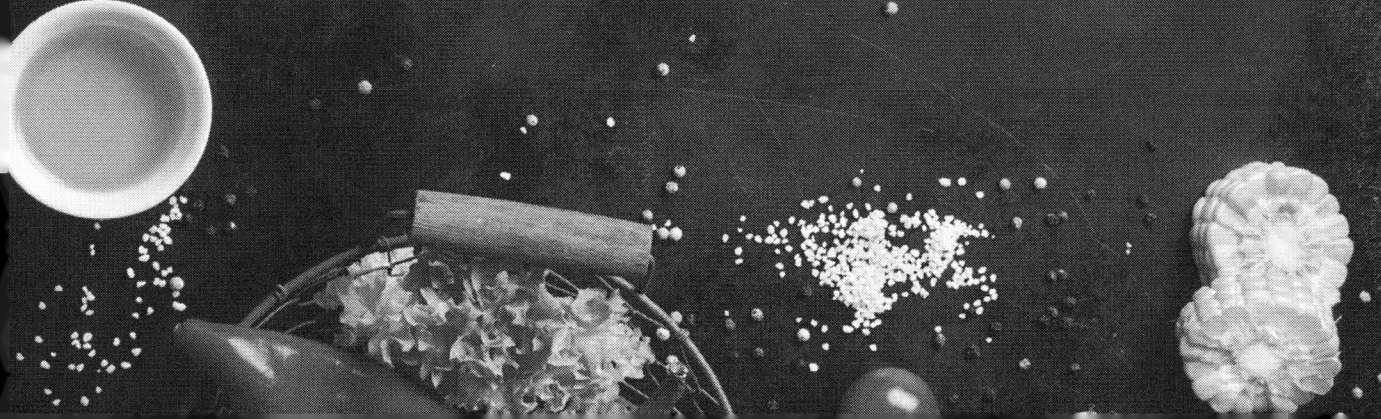

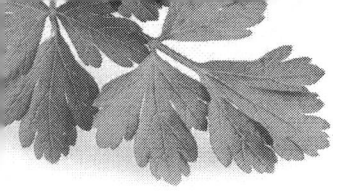

Brownie Batter Fruit Dip

(Prep Time: 5 MIN | Cook Time: N/A | Serves: 8)

Ingredients:

For dip:
1 (14 ounce) can chickpeas (rinsed and drained)
¼ cup cocoa powder
2 tsp calorie-free sweetener
2 tsp vanilla essence
¼ cup almond milk (unsweetened)

Directions:
1. Add all of the ingredients (excluding the almond milk) to a blender and blitz until smooth.
2. Scrape down the sides and with the blender running add the milk a little at a time until you reach your desired consistency.
3. Serve with your favorite NO Points fruits.

Freestyle Points Per Serving: 0

(Calories 80 | Total Fats 2g | Net Carbs: 13g | Protein 4g | Fiber: 1g)

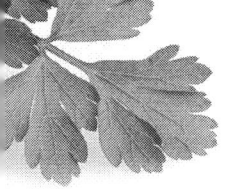

Caramel Pretzel Balls

(Prep Time: 40 MIN | Cook Time: N/A | Serves: 20)

Ingredients:

For balls:

⅓ cup pretzels (crushed
1⅓ cup oats
1 tsp vanilla
2 tbsp mini milk choc chips
¼ cup no added sugar caramel ice cream sauce
¼ cup reduced-fat peanut butter
2½ tbsp honey

Directions:

1. Add all ingredients to a bowl and combine using hands. Chill the mixture for half an hour.
2. Roll 1 tbsp of mixture at a time to create 20 small balls.
3. Enjoy straight away or keep chilled until ready to serve.

Freestyle Points Per Serving: 2

(Calories 70 | Total Fats 2g | Net Carbs: 11g | Protein 1.5g | Fiber: 1g)

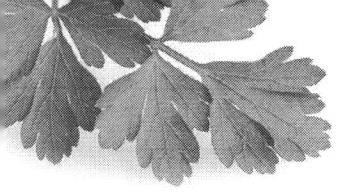

Crunchy Cajun Spiced Chickpeas

(Prep Time: 20 MIN | Cook Time: 40 MIN | Serves: 6)

Ingredients:

For chickpeas:
Nonstick spray
30 ounces canned chickpeas (rinsed, drained, patted dry)

Seasoning:
½ tsp powdered garlic
½ tsp kosher salt
¼ tsp onion powder
¼ tsp black pepper
½ tsp smoked paprika
¼ tsp oregano
¼ tsp cayenne pepper
¼ tsp thyme

Directions:

1. Preheat the main oven to 400 degrees F.
2. Arrange the chickpeas in an even, single layer on a cookie sheet.
3. Place in the oven and bake for half an hour, shaking the cookie sheet every 10 minutes.
4. While the chickpeas cook, add all of the seasoning ingredients to a large bowl and stir to mix.
5. As soon as the chickpeas are cooked, spritz them generously with nonstick spray and tip them into the bowl of seasoning.
6. Toss until the chickpeas are evenly coated. Return the coated chickpeas to the cookie sheet and pop back in the oven for a final 10-12 minutes.
7. After 10-12 minutes, turn the oven off and allow the chickpeas to rest inside for another 10-12 minutes.
8. Take the chickpeas out of the oven and allow to cool before enjoying.

Freestyle Points Per Serving: 3

(Calories 130 | Total Fats 1g | Net Carbs: 16g | Protein 8g | Fiber: 8g)

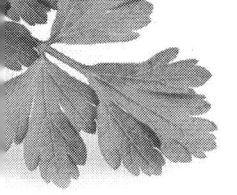

Frozen Yogurt Candy Buttons

(Prep Time: 2 HOUR 5 MIN | Cook Time: N/A | Serves: 6)

Ingredients:

For buttons:

1 (3½) ounce tub fat-free plain Greek yogurt

½ tbsp rainbow sprinkles

Directions:

1. Transfer the yogurt to a Ziploc bag and snip off the corner.
2. 'Pipe' the yogurt onto a cookie sheet in small buttons.
3. Scatter the buttons with sprinkles and freeze for 2 hours before enjoying.

Freestyle Points Per Serving: 1

(Calories 85 | Total Fats 1.5g | Net Carbs: 12g | Protein 5.5g | Fiber: 0g)

SNACKS

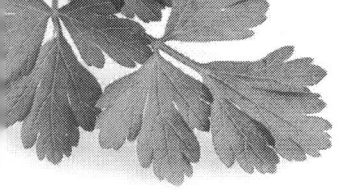

Garlic Breaded Mozzarella Sticks

(Prep Time: 2 HOUR 15 MIN | Cook Time: 10 MIN | Serves: 12)

Ingredients:

For cooking:
Nonstick spray

For mozzarella sticks:
12 string cheese snack sticks (cut in half crosswise)
1 large egg (beaten)
2 tbsp plain flour
¾ tsp powdered garlic
⅔ cup panko breadcrumbs
¼ tsp kosher salt
Pinch black pepper
¾ cup tomato pizza sauce (for dipping)

Directions:

1. Arrange the string cheeses on a plate and pop in the freezer for a couple of hours until solid.
2. Preheat the main oven to 400 degrees F. Cover a baking tray with aluminum foil and spritz with nonstick spray, set to one side.
3. Add the beaten egg to one small bowl. In a second bowl, add the flour. To a third bowl add the powdered garlic, breadcrumbs, kosher salt, and pepper stirring well.
4. Dip each frozen cheese stick first in the flour, then the beaten egg, and finally the seasoned breadcrumbs before arranging on the baking tray. Spritz the coated sticks with nonstick spray.
5. Place in the oven for 5 minutes before flipping over and spritzing again. Bake for a final 5 minutes. Take care not to allow the cheese to melt.
6. Allow the mozzarella sticks to cool for a few minutes before serving with pizza sauce for dipping.

Freestyle Points Per Serving: 2

(Calories 80 | Total Fats 3g | Net Carbs: 5g | Protein 7g | Fiber: 0g)

FREESTYLE 2018

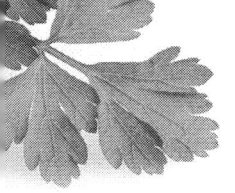

Greek Style Nachos

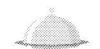 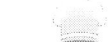

(Prep Time: 5 MIN | Cook Time: 10 MIN | Serves: 2)

Ingredients:

For nachos:

- 2 small whole wheat rounds of pita
- ½ cup grape tomatoes (quartered)
- ¾ cup cucumber (diced)
- 2 tbsp store-bought hummus
- ¼ cup feta cheese (crumbled)

Directions:

1. Preheat the main oven to 375 degrees F.
2. Slice each pita into 8 triangles and arrange on a cookie sheet.
3. Place in the oven and bake for 8-9 minutes until toasted.
4. Divide between two plates and top with an equal amount of tomatoes, cucumber, hummus, and feta. Enjoy.

Freestyle Points Per Serving: 5

(Calories 170 | Total Fats 6g | Net Carbs: 16g | Protein 7.5g | Fiber: 4g)

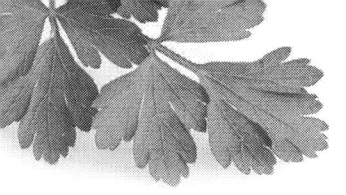

Hawaiian Pizza Cups

(Prep Time: 15 MIN | Cook Time: 25 MIN | Serves: 12)

Ingredients:

For cooking:
Nonstick spray

For pizza cups:
¾ pound Italian hot turkey sausage (without casings)
2 ounces turkey pepperoni (chopped)
1 cup fresh pineapple (peeled, finely chopped)
½ tsp Italian seasoning mix
1 cup tomato pizza sauce
24 wonton wrappers
4 ounces low-fat mozzarella cheese (shredded)

Directions:

1. Preheat the main oven to 375 degrees F. Spritz a 12-hole muffin tin with nonstick spray and set to one side.
2. In a skillet over moderate heat, cook the sausage until brown and fully cooked.
3. Use a wooden spoon to break the sausage up into small pieces as it cooks. Transfer to a large bowl along with the chopped pepperoni, pineapple, seasoning mix, and pizza sauce. Stir well to combine.
4. Arrange one wonton wrapper in each hole of the muffin the tin. Use half of the sausage mixture to spoon on top of each wrapper and sprinkle with half of the cheese.
5. Arrange a second wonton wrapper on top of each cup and gently press down. Top with the remaining sausage mixture and cheese.
6. Place in the oven and bake for just under 20 minutes until hot and golden.
7. Allow to cool a little before serving.

Freestyle Points Per Serving: 3

(Calories 135 | Total Fats 5g | Net Carbs: 11g | Protein 6g | Fiber: 1g)

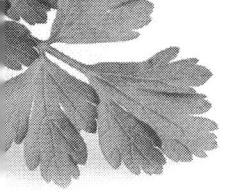

Homemade Potato Chips

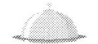

(Prep Time: 10 MIN | Cook Time: 10 MIN | Serves: 2)

Ingredients:

For cooking:
Nonstick spray

For potato chips:
1 (8 ounce) baking potato (very thinly sliced)
½ tsp olive oil
Sea salt

Directions:

1. Line a large plate with parchment and spritz with nonstick spray.
2. Add the sliced potato and olive oil to a Ziploc bag and shake well until coated.
3. Add a generous pinch of salt and shake again.
4. Transfer the potato chips to the plate, arranging in a single layer (work in batches if necessary). Cook in the microwave for 5-10 minutes on a high heat*.
5. Allow to cool for a few minutes before enjoying.

   *Timing will depend on your microwave. Keep checking the potatoes regularly. They are ready when golden and crispy.

Freestyle Points Per Serving: 2

(Calories 85 | Total Fats 1.5g | Net Carbs: 14g | Protein 2g | Fiber: 3g)

SNACKS

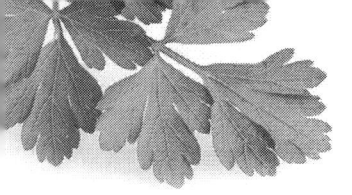

Hot 'n Cheesy Buffalo Chicken Dip

(Prep Time: 10 MIN | Cook Time: 20 MIN | Serves: 12)

Ingredients:

For dip:

- 7 ounces cooked chicken breast (shredded)
- ½ cup hot sauce
- 8 ounces low-fat cream cheese (at room temperature)
- 2 ounces low-fat Cheddar cheese (grated)
- ⅓ cup low-fat bleu cheese dressing

Directions:

1. Preheat the main oven to 350 degrees F.
2. Add all dip ingredients to a large bowl and stir well until combined. Transfer to a 9" pie dish, spreading the mixture out evenly.
3. Place in the oven and bake for 18-20 minutes until bubbly and hot through.
4. Allow to cool for a few minutes before serving with your favorite Zero Point veggies.

Freestyle Points Per Serving: 3

(Calories 105 | Total Fats 7g | Net Carbs: 2g | Protein 8g | Fiber: 0g)

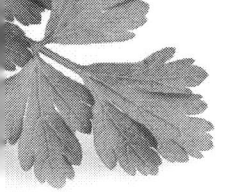

Parmesan Kale Chips

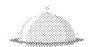

(Prep Time: 5 MIN | Cook Time: 15 MIN | Serves: 6)

Ingredients:

For cooking:
Nonstick spray

For chips:
12 ounces stemless kale (washed, patted dry)
Pinch kosher salt
½ cup Parmesan cheese (shredded)

Directions:

1. Preheat the main oven to 350 degrees F. Spritz two baking sheet with nonstick spray and set to one side.
2. Tear/chop the kale into bite-size pieces and arrange on the baking sheets. Spritz the kale with more nonstick spray and season with kosher salt.
3. Place in the oven and bake for just over 10 minutes, turning the baking sheets halfway through cooking.
4. Remove and sprinkle with the Parmesan, return to the oven for a final 5 minutes until nice and crispy. Allow to cool a little before serving.

Freestyle Points Per Serving: 1

(Calories 50 | Total Fats 3g | Net Carbs: 2.5g | Protein 3.5g | Fiber: 1g)

SNACKS

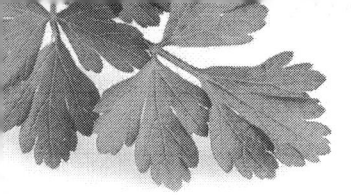

Ranch Style Hummus

(Prep Time: 10 MIN | Cook Time: N/A | Serves: 6)

Ingredients:

For hummus:

½ cup non-fat plain Greek yogurt
1 (15½ ounce) can chickpeas (rinsed, drained)
1 tsp onion powder
1 tsp powdered garlic
1 tsp dill
1 tsp parsley
¼ tsp black pepper
½ tsp sea salt

Directions:

1. Add all hummus ingredients to a blender and blitz for 2-3 minutes until lump-free and smooth.
2. Serve with your favorite Zero Point veggies.

Freestyle Points Per Serving: 0

(Calories 75 | Total Fats 1g | Net Carbs: 9g | Protein 6g | Fiber: 4g)

Soups, Stews & Chillies

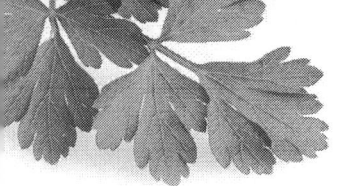

Fiery Caribbean Chicken Stew

(Prep Time: 20 MIN | Cook Time: 35 MIN | Serves: 6)

Ingredients:

For cooking:
1 tsp coconut oil

For chicken:
1 fresh lime
6 chicken thighs (skin removed)
6 chicken drumsticks (skin removed)
1 medium carrot (finely chopped)
2 tsp cornstarch
1½ cups unsweetened light coconut milk
¼ tsp sea salt

For marinade:
1 large tomato (chopped)
4 medium scallions (chopped)
1 large onion (peeled, chopped)
2 cloves garlic (peeled, chopped)
¾ Scotch Bonnet pepper (seeded, membrane removed, chopped)
4 sprigs fresh thyme
2 tbsp low-salt soy sauce

Directions:

1. Squeeze the fresh lime over the chicken.
2. Using clean hands combine the marinade ingredients in a mixing bowl. Add the chicken to the bowl and allow to marinate for a minimum of 60 minutes.
3. Heat the oil in a saucepan over moderately high heat.
4. Take the chicken out of the marinade, reserving the marinade.
5. Add the chicken to the pan and sauté until browned all over.
6. Pour the marinade over the chicken and add the chopped carrots. Stir and cook for approximately 10 minutes.
7. Combine the cornstarch with the light coconut milk and pour into the pan. Continue to cook for 20 minutes.
8. Season to taste, and serve.

Freestyle Points Per Serving: 6

(Calories 235 | Total Fats 9g | Net Carbs: 7g | Protein 27.5g | Fiber: 1.5g)

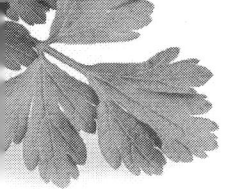

Italian Wedding Soup with Meatballs

(Prep Time: 20 MIN | Cook Time: 40 MIN | Serves: 6)

Ingredients:

For cooking:
3 tsp olive oil

For meatballs:
6 ounce (99%) fat-free ground turkey breast
⅛ tsp garlic powder
1 tbsp Parmesan cheese (freshly grated)
2 tbsp breadcrumbs
¾ tsp Italian seasoning
1 large egg white
1 tbsp skimmed milk

For soup:
½ cup onion (peeled, diced)
2 carrots (diced)
2 cloves garlic (peeled, minced)
Sea salt and black pepper
64 ounces fat-free chicken broth
4 tbsp Parmesan cheese (freshly grated)
½ cup whole wheat orzo (uncooked)
2 cups kale (thinly sliced)

Directions:

1. Add all of the meatball ingredients to a large bowl and combine using clean hands.
2. Roll the mixture into mini meatballs of approximately ¾" diameter. You should yield 30 meatballs in total.
3. In a large pot, over moderate heat, heat 2 tsp of oil. Add the mini meatballs to the pot and while occasionally stirring, cook until browned all over. Transfer to a dish and set to one side.
4. Add the remaining 1 tsp of oil to the pot and continue cooking over moderate heat. Add the onion, followed by the carrots and garlic and season with salt and pepper. Cook, while occasionally stirring for another 4-5 minutes, until the vegetables are fork tender.
5. Pour the chicken broth into the pot and cover with a lid. Bring to boil before removing the lid and adding the mini meatballs, along with the 4 tbsp of Parmesan cheese, orzo, and kale. Stir to incorporate and keep at a boil.
6. Cover the pot and return to moderate heat. Simmer for 12-15 minute until the meatballs and orzo are sufficiently cooked.
7. Serve.

Freestyle Points Per Serving: 3

(Calories 168 | Total Fats 5g | Net Carbs: 15g | Protein 14g | Fiber: 3g)Bottom of Form

SOUPS, STEWS & CHILLIES

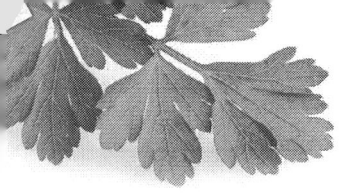

Mexican Chicken Tortilla Soup

(Prep Time: 20 MIN | Cook Time: 4 HOUR | Serves: 8)

Ingredients:

1 pound cooked chicken (shredded)
1 yellow onion (peeled, chopped)
1 (10 ounce) jar enchilada sauce
2 garlic cloves (peeled, minced)
1 (15 ounce) can chopped tomatoes
1 (4 ounce) can green chili peppers (finely chopped)
2 cups cold water
1 (14½ ounce) can chicken broth
10 ounces frozen corn
1 tbsp cilantro (chopped)

Seasoning:

1 tsp chili powder
1 tsp cumin
1 bay leaf
1 tsp sea salt
¼ tsp black pepper

For tortillas:

7 yellow corn tortillas
Canola oil

Directions:

1. Add the shredded chicken, onion, enchilada sauce, garlic, tomatoes, and chili pepper in your slow cooker. Pour in the water along with the chicken broth, and seasoning.
2. Stir in the frozen corn followed by the cilantro.
3. Cover with a tight-fitting lid, and on a low setting, cook for 3-4 hours, on high.
4. Preheat the main oven to 400 degrees F.
5. Lightly brush both sides of the tortillas with canola oil. Cut the tortilla into fine strips and arrange them, in a single layer, on a baking tray.
6. Bake in the oven for between 10-15 minutes, until crisp.
7. Scatter the crisp tortilla strips over the soup and serve.

Freestyle Points Per Serving: 7

(Calories 262 | Total Fats 11g | Net Carbs: 21g | Protein 18g | Fiber: 4g)

FREESTYLE 2018

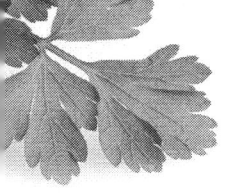

Mixed Vegetable and Lentil Stew

(Prep Time: 15 MIN | Cook Time: 8 HOUR 10 MIN | Serves: 6)

Ingredients:

For vegetables:
2 cups butternut squash (peeled, cubed)
2 cups red potatoes (chopped)
2 cups carrots (chopped)
1½ cups dry lentils
2 cups celery (chopped)
1 medium onion (peeled, diced)
4 garlic cloves (peeled, minced)
8 cups vegetable broth
2 tbsp virgin olive oil
4 cups spinach
½ cup parsley

Seasoning:
2 tsp herbs de Provence
1 tsp smoked paprika
1 tsp kosher salt
Salt and black pepper

Directions:

1. Add the butternut squash, potatoes, carrots, lentils, celery, onion, garlic, broth, and seasoning to a slow cooker, and on low heat, cook for between 7-8 hours.
2. Add approximately a third of the soup to a food blender together with the oil and process until lump free. Return to the slow cooker.
3. Stir in the spinach and parsley and cook for another 6-10 minutes, until the spinach begins to wilt.

Freestyle Points Per Serving: 4

(Calories 320 | Total Fats 5g | Net Carbs: 36g | Protein 16g | Fiber: 19g)

SOUPS, STEWS & CHILLIES

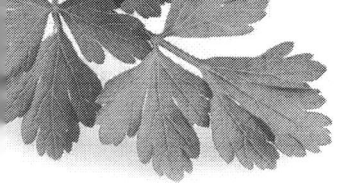

Salmon and Potato Chowder

(Prep Time: 20 MIN | Cook Time: 40 MIN | Serves: 6)

Ingredients:

For chowder:

- 1 red or white onion (peeled, chopped)
- 1 celery stalk (diced)
- ½ red bell pepper (diced)
- 3 garlic cloves
- 2 tbsp fresh thyme (chopped)
- ½ tsp red pepper flakes
- ½ pound potatoes
- 2¾ cups vegetable broth
- ¾ cup frozen corn
- ¼ cup all-purpose flour
- 2½ cups skim milk
- ¾ tsp salt
- ½ tsp ground pepper
- 1¼ pounds fresh salmon (cut into 1" pieces)
- ¼ cup flat leaf parsley (minced)

For cooking:

- 1 tbsp olive oil

Directions:

1. Over moderate heat, in a deep pot, add the oil.
2. Add the onion, followed by the celery, and bell pepper, and cook for 4-5 minutes.
3. Add the garlic along with the thyme, and red pepper flakes, and cook for 60 seconds.
4. Add the potatoes and pour in the vegetable broth. Bring to boil, before reducing the heat a little and simmering until the potatoes are fork tender, approximately 15 minutes.
5. Stir in the frozen corn and simmer for a couple of minutes.
6. In a mixing bowl, whisk the flour with the milk until lump free and add to the pan along with the salt and pepper. Cook, while whisking for several minutes until nice and thick.
7. Add the salmon and cook for another several minutes until the fish is cooked through.
8. Stir in the parsley and serve.

Freestyle Points Per Serving: 4

(Calories 325 | Total Fats 11.5g | Net Carbs: 21.5g | Protein 31.5g | Fiber: 2.5g)

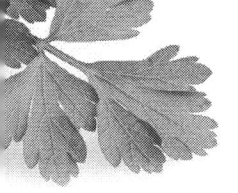

South American Beef and Beer Stew

(Prep Time: 15 MIN | Cook Time: 2 HOUR 10 MIN | Serves: 5)

Ingredients:

For cooking:
2 tsp virgin olive oil

Seasoning:
Sea salt
½ tsp cumin
¼ tsp annatto seasoning
1 bay leaf

For stew:
1 cup scallions (chopped)
3 garlic cloves (peeled, minced)
2 tomatoes (chopped)
2 tbsp cilantro (minced)
1½ pounds best round beef stew (cut into small chunks)
⅓ cup light beer
⅓ cup water
10 ounces baby red potatoes (quartered)

Directions:

1. In a large pot, over moderate heat, heat the oil.
2. Add the scallions along with the garlic and fry for between 2-3 minutes.
3. Add the tomatoes followed by the cilantro. Cook for a couple of minutes, while continually stirring.
4. Add the beef and pour in the light beer and water followed by the seasoning.
5. Cover the pot with a tight-fitting lid and on low heat, simmer for 1½ hours.
6. Check to see if the beef falls apart easily and if it doesn't, continue cooking for another 4-6 minutes.
7. Add the baby potatoes and cook until fork tender, around 20-25 minutes, depending on their size.

Freestyle Points Per Serving: 7

(Calories 193 | Total Fats 5.5g | Net Carbs: 10g | Protein 23g | Fiber: 1.5g)Bottom of Form

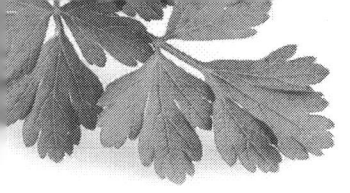

Split Pea and Ham Soup

(Prep Time: 15 MIN | Cook Time: 25 MIN | Serves: 8)

Ingredients:

For cooking:
1 tsp olive oil

For soup:
1 pound dry green split peas
2 carrots (peeled, diced)
1 medium onion (peeled, diced)
¼ cup celery (diced)
2 garlic cloves (peeled, minced)
1 leftover ham bone
6 cups cold water
1 cube bouillon
1 bay leaf
4 ounces ham (diced)
Chives (chopped, to garnish)

Directions:

1. Rinse the peas until cold running water.
2. Add the carrots, onion, celery, and garlic to a pressure cooker, and on a sauté setting, fry in the oil for between 4-5 minutes.
3. Add the leftover ham bone followed by the rinsed peas, cold water, bouillon cube, and bay leaf. Cover and on high pressure, cook for 15 minutes. Allow the pressure to release before opening and removing the ham bone along with the bay leaf. Stir, while the soup thickens as it rests.
4. In a hot frying pan or skillet, sauté the ham to use as a garnish along with the chopped chives.

Freestyle Points Per Serving: 1

(Calories 182 | Total Fats 1.5g | Net Carbs: 24g | Protein 17g | Fiber: 15g) Bottom of Form

FREESTYLE 2018

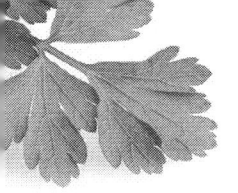

Stracciatella Soup with Spinach and Orzo

(Prep Time: 15 MIN | Cook Time: 20 MIN | Serves: 6)

Ingredients:

7 cups low-sodium chicken broth (divided)
2 large, organic eggs
½ cup Parmesan cheese (freshly grated)
¼ cup flat-leaf parsley (chopped)
4 ounces orzo (uncooked)
6 ounces baby spinach
Salt (to season)
Black pepper (to season)

Directions:

1. Add 6 cups of chicken broth to a pot and bring to boil.
2. In a mixing bowl, combine the remaining cup of broth with the eggs, Parmesan, and parsley, whisk to incorporate.
3. Add the mixture to the boiling broth in the pot and cook for between 3-4 minutes.
4. Add the orzo, cooking for the time indicated by the package instructions.
5. As soon as the orzo is sufficiently cooked, add the baby spinach and mix until it begins to wilt.
6. Remove the pan from the heat. Season with salt and pepper.
7. Ladle the soup into bowls and serve.

Freestyle Points Per Serving: 4

(Calories 127 | Total Fats 4g | Net Carbs: 10g | Protein 10g | Fiber: 1g)Bottom of Form

SOUPS, STEWS & CHILLIES

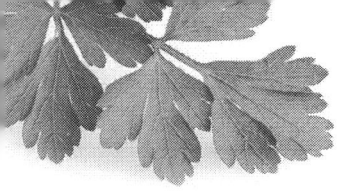

Traditional Minestrone Soup

(Prep Time: 25 MIN | Cook Time: 8 HOUR 15 MIN | Serves: 8)

Ingredients:

For cooking:
2 tsp virgin olive oil

Seasoning:
1 fresh sprig of rosemary
2 bay leaves
2 tbsp fresh basil (chopped)
¼ cup fresh Italian parsley (chopped)
½ tsp sea salt and freshly ground black pepper

For soup:
1 (15 ounce) can navy beans (drained, rinsed)
1 (32 ounce) can reduced-salt chicken broth
½ onion (peeled, chopped)
1 cup carrots (diced)
½ cup celery (diced)
2 cloves garlic (peeled, minced)

1 (28 ounce) can small diced tomatoes
Parmesan cheese rind
8 ounces zucchini (diced)
2 cups fresh spinach (chopped)
2 cups al dente, cooked pasta
Parmesan cheese (to garnish)

Directions:

1. In a food blender, puree the navy beans together with 1 cup of chicken broth.
2. In a large skillet over moderately high heat, add the oil. Add the onion, followed by the carrots, celery, minced garlic and fry until fragrant and tender; approximately 12-15 minutes.
3. Transfer the mixture to a crock pot followed by the remaining chicken broth, tomatoes, pureed navy bean mixture, cheese rind, and seasoning. Cover with a tight-fitting lid and on low, cook for between 6-8 hours.
4. Approximately 45 minutes before the soup is sufficiently cooked, add the zucchini and spinach. Cover with a lid and cook for another 30 minutes. Remove the bay leaves, sprig of rosemary, Parmesan rind, and season to taste.
5. Ladle the soup evenly between 8 bowls. Add ¼ cup of al dente pasta to each bowl and garnish with Parmesan cheese.

Freestyle Points Per Serving: 2

(Calories 190 | Total Fats 3g | Net Carbs: 24g | Protein 9g | Fiber: 8g)

FREESTYLE 2018

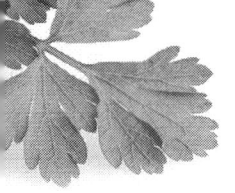

Turkey Chilli Soup

(Prep Time: 15 MIN | Cook Time: 25 MIN | Serves: 9)

Ingredients:

For cooking:
Nonstick spray

For soup:
1⅓ pounds 99% lean ground turkey
1 onion (peeled, chopped)
1 red bell pepper (chopped)
1 (10 ounce) can tomatoes with green chilies
1 (15 ounce) can kidney beans (rinsed, drained)
15 ounces corn
8 ounce tomato sauce
1 (1 ounce) packet low-salt taco seasoning
16 ounces fat-free refried beans
2½ cups low-salt chicken stock

Directions:

1. Lightly spritz a large pot with nonstick spray. Add the ground turkey and over moderate heat, brown all over, using a wooden spoon to break up the meat.
2. When sufficiently cooked, add the onions followed by the peppers and cook for between 2-3 minutes.
3. Add the tomatoes, together with the beans, corn, tomato sauce, taco seasoning, refried beans, and stock. Bring to a boil, cover with a tight-fitting lid and simmer for between 12-15 minutes.
4. Serve the soup with your preferred toppings.

Freestyle Points Per Serving: 0

(Calories 225 | Total Fats 2g | Net Carbs: 24g | Protein 22g | Fiber: 7.5g)

SOUPS, STEWS & CHILLIES

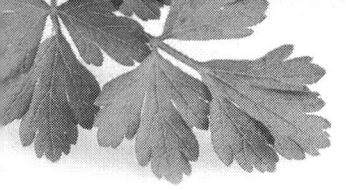

Vegetable and Pumpkin Chilli

(Prep Time: 30 MIN | Cook Time: 1 HOUR 10 MIN | Serves: 10)

Ingredients:

For cooking:
2 tsp virgin olive oil

Seasoning:
1 tbsp chili powder
1 tsp ground cinnamon
2 tsp sea salt
⅛ tsp ground cloves
¼ tsp cayenne pepper
½ tsp ground nutmeg

For topping:
2 small, ripe avocado (peeled, pitted, diced)
5 green onions (finely sliced)
5 tbsp light sour cream
10 tbsp reduced-fat Cheddar cheese (shredded)
2 ounces tortilla chips (crumbled)
Cilantro (chopped, to garnish)

For chili:
1 onion (peeled, diced)
2 large garlic cloves (peeled, crushed)
1 jalapeno (seeded, membrane removed, minced)
2 tbsp fresh ginger (finely minced)
4 Portobello mushrooms (stemmed, wiped clean, cut into cubes)
2 large carrots (diced into ½" cubes)
2 cups frozen corn
2 (14 ounce) cans fire roasted diced tomatoes
1 (14 ounce) can pumpkin puree
1 (14 ounce) can black beans (drained, rinsed)
2 cups low-salt vegetable stock

Directions:

1. Place a large pot over moderately high heat and add the oil.
2. Add the diced onion followed by the garlic, jalapeno, and ginger. Fry until the vegetables are fork tender; this will take between 3-5 minutes.
3. Add the mushrooms and carrots, cook while occasionally stirring for 5-6 minutes.
4. Next, add the seasoning and stir very well.
5. Add the frozen corn, together with the fire roasted tomatoes, pumpkin, black beans and vegetable stock, mixing well to combine.
6. Cover the pot, and reduce the heat to moderate to low, while occasionally stirring, simmer for between 45-50 minutes.
7. As soon as the carrots are tender, remove the pot from the heat and serve with the fresh toppings.

Freestyle Points Per Serving: 2

(Calories 232 | Total Fats 7g | Net Carbs: 26g | Protein 7g | Fiber: 9g)Bottom of Form

Veggies & Vegetarian

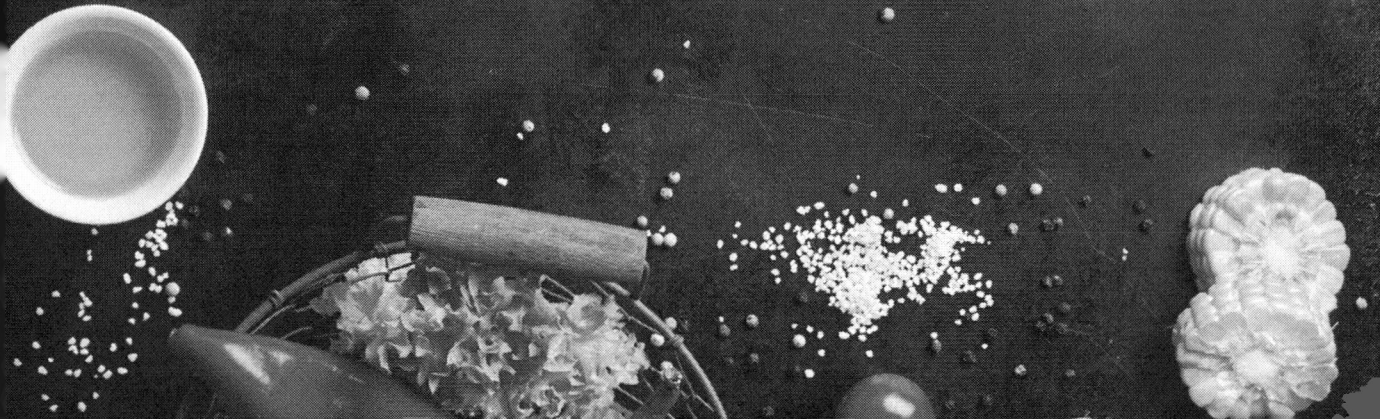

Blueberry and Fresh Corn Salad with Lime Honey Dressing

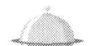

(Prep Time: 10 MIN | Cook Time: 10 MIN | Serves: 4)

Ingredients:

For dressing:
1 tbsp olive oil
1 tbsp freshly squeezed lime juice
¼ tsp sea salt
½ tbsp honey
⅛ tsp cumin
¼ tsp black pepper

For salad:
3 ears corn
1 cup fresh blueberries
¼ cup red onion (peeled, finely chopped)
¼ cup fresh cilantro (roughly chopped)
½ jalapeno (seeded, finely chopped)

Directions:

1. Add all dressing to a small bowl and stir to combine, set aside.
2. Grill the corn ears for 8-9 minutes, turning every so often, until lightly brown. Slice the corn kernels from the cob and add to a serving bowl along with the remaining salad ingredients tossing to combine.
3. Drizzle the dressing over the salad and toss again. Serve.

Freestyle Points Per Serving: 2

(Calories 125 | Total Fats 4g | Net Carbs: 19g | Protein 3g | Fiber: 3g)

FREESTYLE 2018

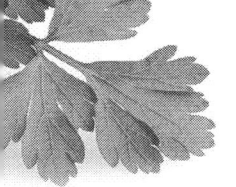

Brie and Pear Grilled Cheese Sandwiches

(Prep Time: 10 MIN | Cook Time: 6 MIN | Serves: 2)

Ingredients:

For sandwiches:

2 tbsp low-calorie butter

4 slices reduced-calorie whole wheat bread

2 ounces rindless Brie (thinly sliced)

½ ounce fresh arugula

½ large, ripe pear (thinly sliced)

1 tsp organic honey

Directions:

1. Butter each slice of bread on one side only.
2. Place two of the slices, non-buttered side up, in a skillet and arrange the sliced Brie, arugula, and pear on top. Drizzle each slice with ½ tsp honey and top with the remaining bread slices, non-buttered side down.
3. Put the skillet over moderate heat and cook for 3 minutes before carefully flipping and cooking for another 3 minutes.
4. Slice and serve.

Freestyle Points Per Serving: 9

(Calories 280 | Total Fats 16g | Net Carbs: 24g | Protein 10g | Fiber: 4g)

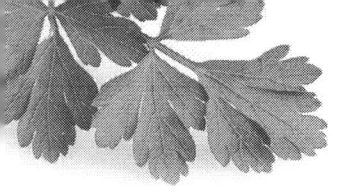

Broccoli Parmigianno

(Prep Time: 10 MIN | Cook Time: 30 MIN | Serves: 4)

Ingredients:

For parmigiano:

1 medium bunch broccoli and stems
6 garlic cloves (peeled, smashed)
2 tbsp virgin olive oil
½ tsp sea salt
1 cup store-bought marinara sauce
½ cup mozzarella cheese (shredded)

Directions:

1. Preheat the main oven to 450 degrees F.
2. Trim and discard approximately 1" off the broccoli stems. Slice each stalk in half across their length until you have a total of 4 pieces.
3. Arrange the broccoli together with the cloves of garlic on a 9x13" baking dish and lightly drizzle both sides of the broccoli with oil. Season each side with sea salt. Place in the preheated oven and roast, cut side facing upwards, for approximately 8-10 minutes, or until the broccoli is gently browned on the bottom. Flip the broccoli and garlic over and roast until tender, crisp and gently browned, this will take another 8-10 minutes.
4. Pour the sauce over the broccoli and top with mozzarella. Return to the oven and bake for another 10 minutes, until the cheese melts and the dish is sufficiently hot.
5. Serve and enjoy.

Freestyle Points Per Serving: 3

(Calories 168 | Total Fats 10.5g | Net Carbs: 8g | Protein 3g | Fiber: 5g)

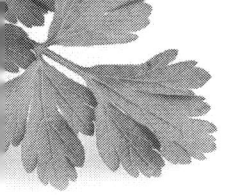

Corn and Zucchini Frittata with Cheese

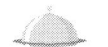

(Prep Time: 20 MIN | Cook Time: 35 MIN | Serves: 6)

Ingredients:

For cooking:
1 tbsp light butter
Nonstick spray

For vegetables:
1 cup fresh corn kernels
1 cup zucchini (thinly sliced)
Salt and pepper (to season)

For eggs:
8 large, organic eggs
⅓ cup fat-free plain Greek yogurt
¾ tsp sea salt
¼ tsp black pepper
1 tbsp chives (diced)
¼ cup fresh basil (sliced)
2 ounces sharp Cheddar cheese (shredded)

Directions:

1. Preheat the main oven to 350 degrees F.
2. Over moderately low heat, melt the butter in a 10" skillet. Add the kernels along with the zucchini and gently stir to coat the vegetables with the melted butter. Season with a pinch of salt and a dash of pepper. Cook, while regularly stirring for 5-7 minutes.
3. In the meantime, while the vegetables cook, whisk together all of the egg ingredients.
4. As soon as the corn and zucchini are sufficiently cooked, transfer them both to the bowl containing the eggs and stir to combine.
5. Generously coat the skillet with nonstick spray.
6. Pour the egg mixture into the skillet and on moderate heat, cook until the outside edges of the frittata become opaque, this will take between 5-7 minutes.
7. Transfer the skillet to the preheated oven and cook until the very center is set; 15-18 minutes.
8. Set to one side to cool for 4-5 minutes before serving.

Freestyle Points Per Serving: 2

(Calories 167 | Total Fats 11g | Net Carbs: 4g | Protein 13g | Fiber: 1g)

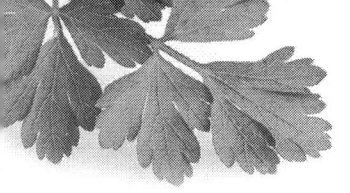

Golden Cauliflower Nuggets

(Prep Time: 20 MIN | Cook Time: 20 MIN | Serves: 6)

Ingredients:

For cooking:
Nonstick spray

For cauliflower:
30 cauliflower florets (5 per serving)
3 large, organic eggs (beaten)

For coating:
1¼ cups whole wheat breadcrumbs (finely ground)
⅓ cup Parmesan cheese (freshly grated)
½ tsp sea salt
Freshly ground black pepper

Directions:

1. Preheat the main oven to 450 degrees F. Spritz a rimmed baking sheet with nonstick spray and set to one side.
2. Add the beaten eggs to a shallow bowl and set aside for a moment.
3. Combine all of the coating ingredients and divide evenly into two bowls.
4. Using cold water, lightly wet one hand, while keeping the second hand perfectly dry. Using the wet hand, evenly coat a few pieces of cauliflower in the egg mixture, gently shaking off any excess mixture.
5. Next, drop the egg-coated cauliflower into one bowl of the coating mixture.
6. With your dry hand, scatter some breadcrumbs from the second bowl of coating mixture on the top of the florets.
7. Transfer the coated florets to the baking sheet and repeat the process until you run out of crumbs. By using more than one bowl, you will prevent soggy breadcrumbs.
8. Lightly spritz the florets with nonstick spray and bake in the oven until fork tender, this will take between 8-10 minutes, flip the florets over and cook for another 8-10 minutes.
9. Serve.

Freestyle Points Per Serving: 3

(Calories 159 | Total Fats 5.5g | Net Carbs: 14g | Protein 10g | Fiber: 5g)

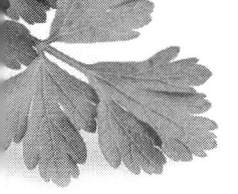

Indian Potato Cauliflower Curry

(Prep Time: 10 MIN | Cook Time: 35 MIN | Serves: 6)

Ingredients:

For spice paste:

1" chunk fresh ginger (peeled, grated)
2 garlic cloves (peeled, minced)
½ tsp red pepper flakes
2 tsp cumin
1 tbsp coriander
2 tsp turmeric
2 tbsp canola oil
½ tsp sea salt

For curry:

1 cauliflower (cut into florets)
1½ pounds potatoes (peeled, cubed)
1¼ cups water
½ cup cilantro (roughly chopped, for garnish)

Directions:

1. Combine all spice paste ingredients in a small bowl and stir until well combined and transfer to a saucepan over low heat.
2. Cook the paste for 5-6 minutes until fragrant and then add the cauliflower florets and potato. Increase the heat to moderate and cook while stirring for 3 minutes.
3. Pour in the water and bring to a simmer. Cover with a lid and cook for half an hour until the veggies are tender.
4. Garnish with cilantro and serve.

Freestyle Points Per Serving: 4

(Calories 135 | Total Fats 5g | Net Carbs: 17.4g | Protein 3g | Fiber: 4g)

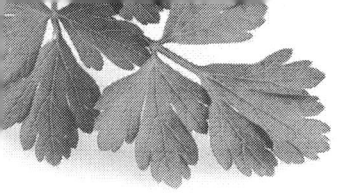

Lemon Avocado Toast with Chia Seeds

(Prep Time: 10 MIN | Cook Time: 5 MIN | Serves: 2)

Ingredients:

For kale:
1 cup stemless kale (shredded)
Juice from ¼ medium lemon
1 tsp olive oil
⅛ tsp kosher salt

For avocado mash:
½ small ripe avocado (pitted, peeled, mashed)
Pinch kosher salt
Pinch black pepper
Juice from ¼ medium lemon

For toast:
4 (1 ounce) slices multigrain bread (toasted)
½ small ripe avocado (pitted, peeled, sliced)
⅛ tsp cumin
1 tsp chia seeds

Directions:

1. Add all of the kale ingredients to a small bowl and stir well. Massage the liquid into the leaves for 60 seconds. Set to one side for a moment.
2. Add all of the avocado mash ingredients to a second small bowl and stir until well combined.
3. Spread the avocado mash equally onto the four toasted bread slices. Top each with an equal amount of sliced avocado, followed by kale, and a sprinkling of cumin and chia seeds. Serve straight away.

Freestyle Points Per Serving: 8

(Calories 300 | Total Fats 14g | Net Carbs: 26g | Protein 11g | Fiber: 10g)

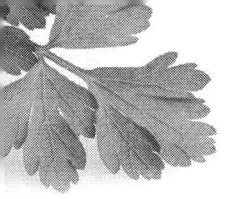

Quinoa and Squash Salad with Citrus Dressing

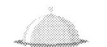

(Prep Time: 10 MIN | Cook Time: 25 MIN | Serves: 5)

Ingredients:

For salad:

1 pound raw butternut squash (peeled, cut into ½" cubes)
2 tsp olive oil
Sea salt
3 cups quinoa (cooked, room temperature)
2 ounces goat cheese (crumbled)
1 tbsp fresh parsley (minced)

For dressing:

2 tsp virgin olive oil
1 tbsp freshly squeezed orange juice
1 tbsp freshly squeezed lemon juice
1 tbsp apple cider vinegar
1 tsp runny honey

Directions:

1. Preheat the main oven to 400 degrees F.
2. Toss the cubes of squash with 2 tsp of oil and scatter with sea salt.
3. In a single layer, arrange the squash on a baking sheet and bake for 25 minutes.
4. Remove from the oven and set aside to cool for several minutes.
5. As soon as the squash is sufficiently cooled, transfer it to a bowl. Add the quinoa and stir in the crumbled goat cheese along with the minced parsley.
6. In a smaller bowl, combine the dressing ingredients, and stir until incorporated.
7. Pour the dressing over the quinoa mixture and stir until evenly coated.
8. Serve either chilled or at room temperature.

Freestyle Points Per Serving: 6

(Calories 250 | Total Fats 10g | Net Carbs: 32g | Protein 8g | Fiber: 4g)

VEGGIES & VEGETARIAN

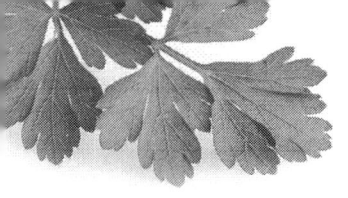

Simple Caesar Salad

(Prep Time: 10 MIN | Cook Time: N/A | Serves: 5)

Ingredients:

For dressing:
⅓ cup fat-free plain Greek yogurt
¼ cup low-fat mayo
1 tbsp red wine vinegar
2 tsp Dijon mustard
1 tsp Worcestershire sauce

For salad:
10 cups romaine lettuce (shredded)
30 Caesar croutons (any brand)
2½ tbsp Parmesan cheese (freshly grated, divided)

Directions:

1. Add all dressing ingredients to a small bowl and stir to combine, set aside.
2. Add 2 cups of shredded romaine lettuce to 5 salad bowls. Top each bowl with 2 tbsp of the dressing and mix gently to coat the lettuce.
3. Scatter 6 croutons on top of each bowl and garnish with ½ tbsp of Parmesan cheese. Serve.

Freestyle Points Per Serving: 2

(Calories 223 | Total Fats 8g | Net Carbs: 28g | Protein 9g | Fiber: 2g)

FREESTYLE 2018

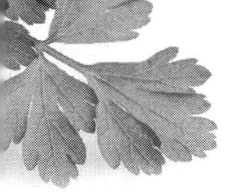

Vegetable Chow Mein

(Prep Time: 10 MIN | Cook Time: 15 MIN | Serves: 4)

Ingredients:

For cooking:
Nonstick spray

For noodles:
4 ounces fresh yaki-soba noodles
2 stalks celery (chopped)
1 yellow onion (peeled, finely chopped)
4 cups cabbage (shredded)

For sauce:
4 garlic cloves (peeled, minced)
¼ cup soy sauce
1 tbsp brown sugar
¼ tsp black pepper
2 tsp fresh ginger (peeled, minced)

Directions:

1. Soak the noodles in boiling water for 2 minutes until tender.
2. In the meantime, whisk together all of the sauce ingredients and set to one side for a moment.
3. To a skillet over moderately high heat, add the oil and sauté the celery and onion for 3 minutes before adding the cabbage and cooking for another 2 minutes.
4. Add the noodles to the skillet along with the set-aside sauce. Stir well and cook for a final few minutes before serving.

Freestyle Points Per Serving: 4

(Calories 140 | Total Fats 4g | Net Carbs: 18g | Protein 4g | Fiber: 5g)

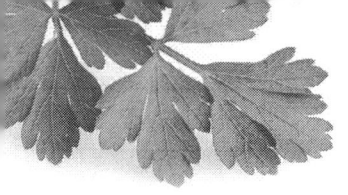

Vegetable Tots

(Prep Time: 8 MIN | Cook Time: 25 MIN | Serves: 5)

Ingredients:

For cooking:

Nonstick spray

For tots:

¼ cup carrots (sliced)
2 cups broccoli florets
¼ small onion
½ cup zucchini (chopped)
2 large, organic eggs
¾ cup panko breadcrumbs
½ tsp salt
⅓ cup roasted garlic hummus

Directions:

1. Preheat the main oven to 400 degrees F. Using aluminum foil, line a baking sheet and spritz with nonstick spray.
2. Add the carrots and broccoli to a microwave-safe bowl and cover with a sheet of damp kitchen towel. Microwave on high for 2 minutes.
3. Transfer to a food blender along with the onion and zucchini. Pulse, several times until the veggies are minced.
4. Transfer the minced vegetables to the bowl and combine with the eggs, breadcrumbs, salt, and hummus. Stir until incorporated.
5. Using a rounded tbsp of vegetable mixture at a time, use clean hands to form into 25 top shapes.
6. Arrange the tots on the prepared baking sheet. Lightly spritz the tots with nonstick spray.
7. Bake in the oven for 20 minutes, flipping halfway through cooking. Serve hot.

Freestyle Points Per Serving: 2

(Calories 116 | Total Fats 5g | Net Carbs: 11g | Protein 3g | Fiber: 2g)

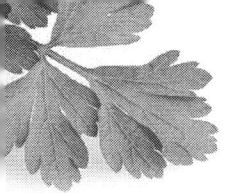

Take Control & Win the War!

For anyone unhappy with their weight, the first step to making a lifestyle change is always the most challenging.

In reading this, you have made a conscious decision, just as Freestyle founder Jean Nidetch did nearly 60 years ago, to make changes for a healthier, happier you!

By following the proven and successful Weight Watcher Freestyle Program, you are well on the way to not only winning the battle against those unwanted pounds but the war!

Just remember these 5 simple guidelines:
- NO Points don't need to be measured, weighed or tracked, so make the most of them!
- Rollover points can help you enjoy life to the full, guilt-free
- Track all foods with a Smart Point value
- Make yourself familiar with the new NO Points foods
- Avoid boredom by getting creative in the kitchen with our exciting sweet and savory recipes

Thank you for taking the time to read this book, and we wish you every success.

Don't forget; eat well, and live longer.

Jean Nidetch lived life to the full until the grand old age of 91, and didn't once top the scales at more than 150 pounds!

SOPHIA LEE

Made in the USA
Middletown, DE
29 September 2018